CW01647169

Access the management to[illegible]

the following web page:

http://www.servet.es/management/peremercader/

Scratch here to find your password.

M1SP-3W0U-NQ55

MANAGEMENT SOLUTIONS FOR VETERINARY PRACTICES

Pere Mercader (DVM, MBA, DEA)

Caution:
Veterinary science is subject to constant evolution and change, as are pharmacology and other sciences. Therefore, it is the absolute responsibility of the veterinary practitioner, drawing on his/her professional experience, to determine and check the dosage, method, period of administration and the possible contraindications of the treatments applied to each patient.

Neither the Publisher nor the authors accept responsibility for any damages that may result to people, animals or property as a consequence of the use or incorrect application of the information contained in this work.

This book has been published originally in spanish under the title:
Soluciones de gestión para clínicas veterinarias

ISBN spanish edition: 978-84-92569-06-9

For this english edition:

Andador Palacio de Larrinaga, 2
50013 Zaragoza

Translators/Proofreaders:
Sally Coleman BA (Hons), AMA, MCIM, CELTA

Design and layout:
Servet editorial - Grupo Asís Biomedia, S.L.
www.servet.es

Printing:
mccgraphics
Planta Elkar
Larrondo Beheko Etorbidea, Edif. 4
48180 Loiu (Bizkaia)

ISBN: 978-84-92569-58-8
D.L.: BI-1934/2011

Printed in Spain

MANAGEMENT SOLUTIONS FOR VETERINARY PRACTICES

Pere Mercader (DVM, MBA, DEA)

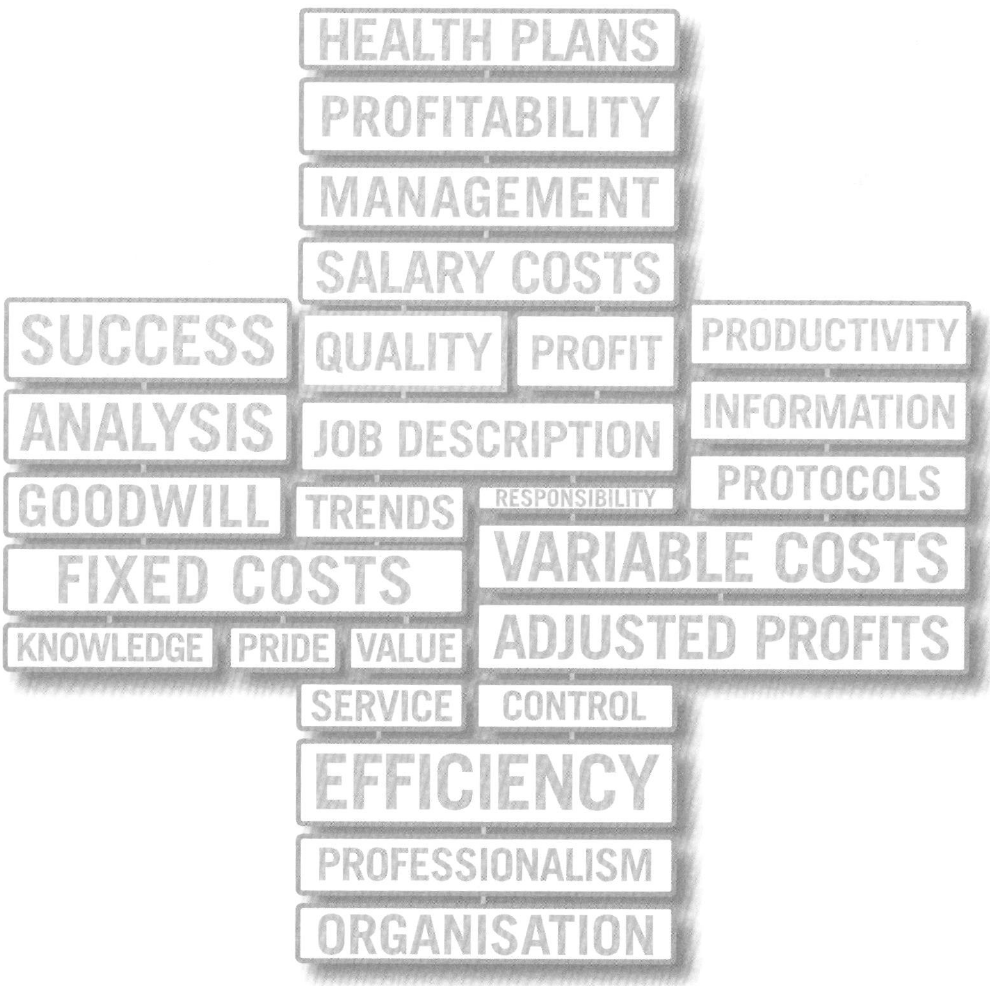

ABOUT THE AUTHOR

Pere Mercader is a graduate in veterinary science from the Universidad Autonoma de Barcelona and also has a Masters in Business Administration MBA (IESE) and a Diploma of Advanced Studies in Economics and Business (Universidad Pompeu Fabra).

He worked for 10 years in executive positions in marketing and market research for a multinational company in the companion animal sector. From 2001 he has been a management consultant specialising in veterinary practice management for several veterinary hospitals in Spain and Portugal. He collaborated with AVEPA (Spanish Small Animal Veterinary Association) to found the IVEE (Veterinary Institute of Economic Studies). He has developed projects which include studies on the profitability of Spanish veterinary practices, price studies on veterinary practice services, studies on pet owners´ perceptions of veterinary surgeons, etc.

He has taught courses and given seminars on practice management in more than twenty countries in America, Asia and Europe. He is the first Spanish member of the Association of Veterinary Practice Managment Consultants and Advisors (AVPMCA). He has also been Associate Lecturer in the Department of Economics and Business at the Universidad of Pompeu Fabra. He is a lecturer and coordinator for the modules on Marketing and Strategy on the Masters course in Administration and Management of Veterinary Practices of the AVEPA-UAB, the first European programme of this kind.

Pere is also a founder member and director of VMS – Veterinary Management Studies (www.estudiosveterinarios.com), an economic research company specialising in Spanish veterinary practices.

PREFACE

In my experience, small animal veterinary surgeons in many countries have a remarkably similar vision of their profession and about money. I have dedicated the last seven years of my professional career to providing management advice to veterinary practices. During that time I have met hundreds of vets; mainly Spanish, but also Portuguese, French, Greek, North American, Central American... I met them at their own practices, during scientific congresses and at management conferences. Despite the cultural and economic differences between their countries, it has never failed to amaze me how similar their concerns are. Every time I speak with one of them about the problems of the profession, about their business perspective or about their relationship with both clients and employees, I always hear the same things.

My experiences with those vets has led me to discover a warm-hearted group of people, passionate about their profession, always eager to learn, dedicated and generous to a fault. They are an endearing and admirable group of people who, in my humble opinion, are incomparable with any other profession. However they have also often shown me that they are a profession with low self-esteem, with a guilt complex when defending decent earnings in front of their clients, with less dedication to their clients and employees than to their patients, with poor communication skills and with an unhealthy tendency towards fatalism and blaming others for all their problems. The result of this painful combination is an inadequate level of financial reward and social prestige which is particularly unfair considering the enormous level of personal and professional sacrifice demanded by this profession. This is reflected in the fact that I know few veterinary surgeons that want their children to follow in their footsteps.

Robert Kennedy said: “Some men see what has happened and ask: “Why? I prefer to think about things that have not happened and ask: “Why not?”. If Robert Kennedy had been a vet, instead of spending his time whining about the misfortunes of the profession he would have been wondering why it is not possible to combine good medicine with a reasonable financial return and a decent quality of life. This book is my small tribute to this wonderful profession and an attempt to make a small contribution to find a way so that, in a few years time, these same professionals will want their children to someday become vets.

ACKNOWLEDGEMENTS

I am deeply grateful to each and every one of the vets who have trusted in my professional services over the years. I am indebted to them as, without exception, I have learnt something from each of them. I also want to thank those vets who, in a generous and altruistic way, share their ideas and experiences in the management field with other colleagues. They play an important role in the dissemination of a "new management culture" in veterinary practices. Finally, I want to express my appreciation and thanks to AVEPA (Spanish Small Animal Veterinary Association) for having fought against all odds for the improvement of the profession in all respects and not just from a clinical perspective.

INTRODUCTION

This book is not intended to be either an academic textbook or an exhaustive study on all the different areas of practice management. It is rather a compendium of the experiences of a consultant over ten years in the field. The models and methods discussed here are a homogeneous mix of some (the minority) of my own ideas, adaptations of ideas from other authors and consultants and the rest are adaptions of good practice intuitively designed by my own clients. I have always intended to acknowledge the source of these ideas and apologise in advance for the omissions that will have inevitably been made.

Another important point to clarify concerns the sale of drugs by practices and the way this data is used in some of the financial models in the book. These examples are designed solely to aid understanding of the financial concepts described in the text, irrespective of the obvious duty of the veterinary surgeon to respect the relevant laws in force in each country.

This book has been structured in such way as to allow each chapter to be read independently of the others. However, by way of advice, it is suggested to start by reading chapters 1 and 2, as they provide the framework for the practice management model developed in the subsequent chapters. These chapters explain the fundamentals of practice management and analyse the role of the practice manager.

Chapters 3 and 4 have a financial content and will be best appreciated by those inclined to quantify things. In these chapters the concept of profitability will be analysed and a model for the valuation of a veterinary practice proposed.

If a reader would have time to read just one chapter, this would have to be chapter 5. This chapter is a financial reflexion on how to charge for veterinary services.

Chapter 6 is dedicated to human resources, the "big headache" of most veterinary practice owners. It is a never ending subject and therefore impossible to be comprehensively covered in a single chapter. Some practical examples of the tools most commonly used in modern team management are presented here.

Chapters 7 and 8 will be the favourite areas for lovers of marketing. The first of them is focused around client orientation and in creating a sense of value for our services. The second, of a more technical nature, provides specific "ready to use" examples of client survey templates.

Finally, chapter 9 is devoted to a strategic area of growth for most veterinary practices: preventative medicine.

The book is supplemented with management tools to download which aim to assist the reader to implement some of the ideas discussed here. These tools are templates and forms that, once completed with the information from the reader's own practice, will help to interpret the real situation in their business.

The tool "thermometer of management quality" is an auditing device to see if the practice is being well managed, taking as a reference whether the 20 good practices recommended for service business have been implemented or not.

The tool "the key management indicator calculator" will use your own data to generate a number of results to indicate the business health of your practice.

The tool "profitability thermometer" tries to reflect as realistically as possible the profit of the practice based on financial data supplied by the reader.

The tool "calculator of cost per minute of the vet´s time" calculates the cost to the business of each minute that a vet spends with a client, using data from the reader's veterinary practice. This is key data when setting professional salaries.

The tool "satisfaction survey analyser" proposes a ready-to-use format for client satisfaction surveys. It also allows you to input the responses of up to 100 clients and automatically generate graphs of the results analyses.

INDEX OF CONTENTS

Success factors
for a veterinary practice:
Good management practice

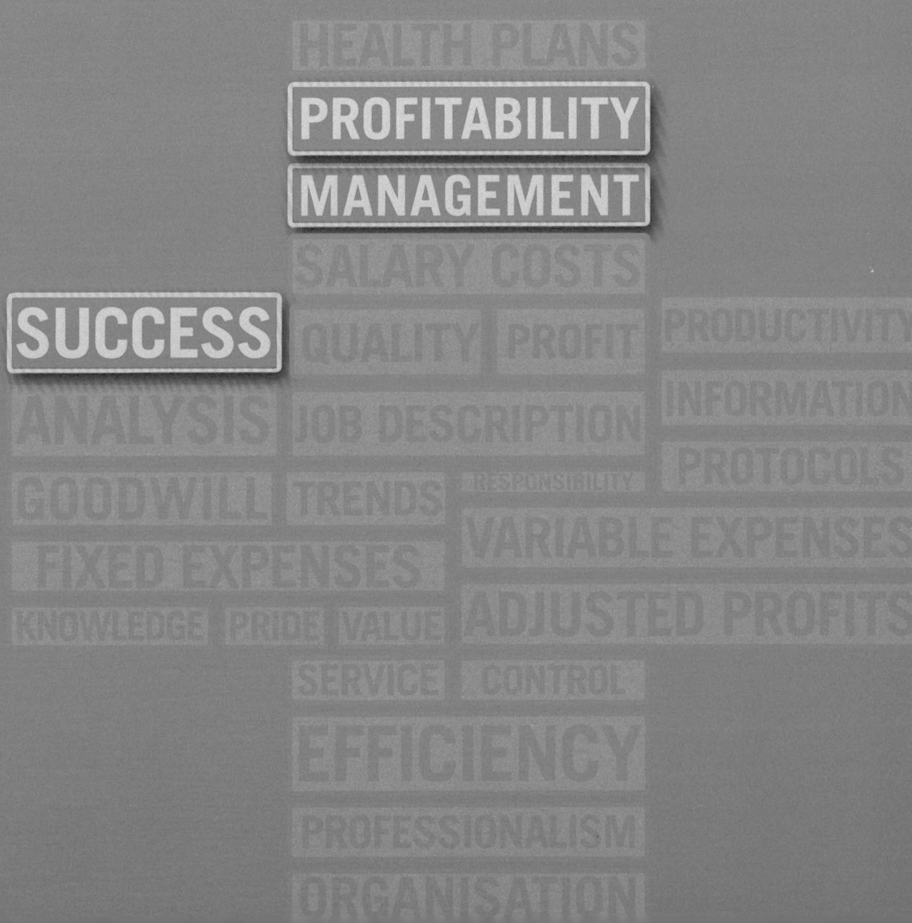

1

What does the profitability of a veterinary practice depend upon?

When the financial results of companies are analysed, important differences can be seen in the profitability achieved. This variability is also evident in the case of businesses of a similar size and that undertake their activities in the same sector, as in the case of veterinary practices.

Why do some veterinary practices that earn 3 million euros and make a profit of 25% of their turnover, coexist alongside other practices that generate less than 100,000 euros and are not even able to pay the owner a salary at the going market rate? What factors are responsible for these fluctuations in profitability?

We need to distinguish between two kinds of factors; those that are uncontrollable or difficult to control by the owner of the business, and those that enter into the sphere of decision-making[1].

Uncontrollable factors or those difficult to control by the owner of the business

- How long the veterinary practice has been in existence.
- Location of the veterinary practice.
- Other competitors in the area (ratio between pets and veterinary practices).
- Owner's gender.

Factors controllable by the owner of the business

- Use of good business management practices.
- Level of economic and financial knowledge.

Uncontrollable factors or those difficult to control by the owner of the veterinary practice

Amongst the uncontrollable factors or those difficult to control by the owner we find:

1. How long the veterinary practice has been in existence

The practices that have been set up the longest are usually well established in their area, have a better client base and therefore higher levels of income (and predictably profits).

2. Location of the veterinary practice

Proximity to home is still the second most frequently cited reason given by pet owners for choosing a veterinary practice for the first time. The practices located in areas of high population density and in locations with high visibility and good access start off with an important advantage. The socio-economic level of the area where the practice is located is also important, as the frequency of visits to the vet increases with the level of education of the pet owner[2].

Frequency[1] of visits to the vet

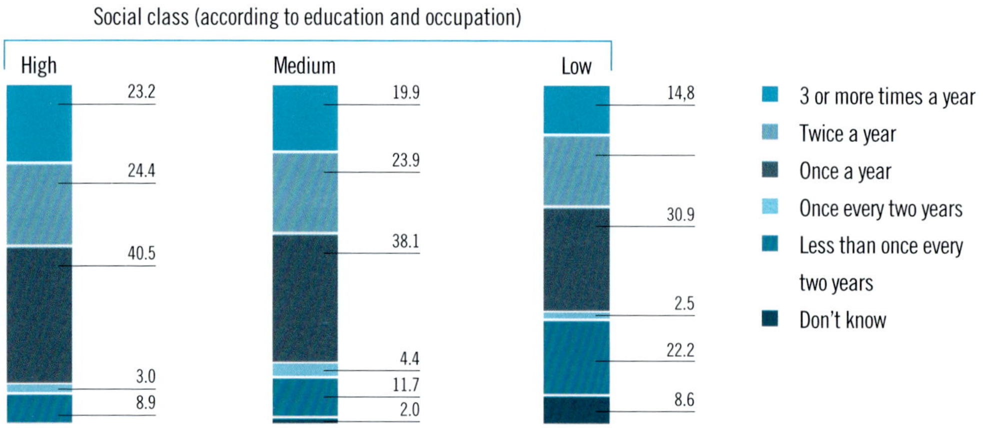

[1] The frequency figures are shown as a percentage.

3. The competition

The ratio of pets registered on the census compared to the number of veterinary practices indicates the competitive dynamics of the profession. To give an example, in a country such as Spain some 5,000 veterinary practices serve the needs of roughly the 6,000,000 dogs and cats that visit the vet. That means around 1,200 potential patients per veterinary practice. This ratio is clearly unfavourable when compared with that existing in other countries like the United States and the United Kingdom. According to these ratios, the competitive environment in Spain is between 3 and 4 times more aggressive than in Britain or the U.S.A. In the author's experience, a veterinary practice is difficult to sustain with less than 1,200 active patient records, which means it needs to have a catchment area with a population of between 7,000 and 8,000 individuals. Those practices located in areas of low competition (with a high number of pets in ratio to the veterinary practices available) will have a better prospect of achieving desirable levels of profitability.

4. The owner's gender

This is a controversial subject, but one that should not be avoided. To date, extensive studies in the United States have demonstrated that the turnover achieved by veterinary practices managed by female professionals is significantly lower. These differences are replicated even when you take the other variables out of the equation such as the location, how long the practice has been established or the hours worked. A financial difference still exists that is not explained by other variables that will undoubtedly need to be investigated in more detail in the future.

Comparison of the professional dynamics between countries

	Spain[1]		USA[2]		Reino Unido[3]	
Number of households	14,270,656		105,000,000		24,700,000	
Number of households with dogs	3,895,889		37,900,000		5,200,000	
Number of households with cats	1,883,727		33,186,000		6,100,000	
% of households with dogs	27.3%		36.1%		21.1%	
% of households with cats	13.2%		31.6%		24.7%	
Average number of dogs per household with dogs	1.2		1.6		1.1	
Average number of cats per household with cats	1.5		2.1		1.6	
Total number of dogs according to the census	4,675,067		61,570,000		6,800,000	
Total number of cats according to the census	2,825,590		70,796,000		9,580,000	
Dogs that go to the vet	4,207,560	90%	58,491,500	95%	6,460,000	95%
Cats that go to the vet	1,836,633	65%	63,716,400	90%	8,622,000	90%
Number of small animal veterinary practices (or predominantly small animals)	5,000		30,000		3,738	
Average number of dogs per veterinary practice	842		1,950		1,728	
Average number of cats per veterinary practice	367		2,124		2,307	
Average number of cats and dogs per veterinary practice	1,209		4,074		4,035	

Sources: 1 **Spain**: Veterindustria, Estudio de cumplimiento AVEPA-Hill´s, Census INE 2001 (revised 2003) own estimations.
2 **USA**: AVMA Pt Census 2001 and Dennis MacCurnin.
3 **UK**: RCVS annual report, PFMA (2004) and John Sheridan.

Factors controllable by the owner of the veterinary practice

There are however another series of controllable factors that equally affect the profitability of the veterinary practice and over which the owner themselves has the capacity to decide. In particular, the use of so-called good business management practices. They are a series of methods, habits and techniques commonly observed in the most successful small and medium-sized service companies. Some of these have been tested in practice[3], whilst others are common knowledge amongst consultants and specialist managers.

At this point a brief introduction to 20 of these good management practices will be made, those that in the author´s experience are more applicable to the idiosyncrasies of the small animal veterinary practice. Over the remaining chapters, a more detailed study will be made covering the analysis and practical use of these methodologies.

20 GOOD MANAGEMENT PRACTICES FOR A PROFITABLE VETERINARY PRACTICE

GOOD PRACTICE 1

Regular review and interpretation of the practice´s financial results

- Do we have a consistent format to record and analyse the income and expenditure of our business?
- Do we carry it out monthly or at least quarterly?
- Do we analyse the trends over time, comparing the results for that period with those of the same period the year before?
- Do we know and monitor our level of debt?
- Do we control our ability to meet our payment obligations?
- Do we calculate our solvency and liquidity ratios?
- Do we measure our working capital needs?

GOOD PRACTICE 2

A well-defined pricing policy

- Have we calculated the costs of our main services and are we sure that we are not losing money with our current list of prices?
- Have we defined how often, and with what criteria, our price list is updated?
- Do we monitor and chase debtors?
- Have we quantified our discounts?
- Is it well defined in the clinic when, who, why and to whom a discount can be given?
- Have we discussed and agreed with our team what arguments to give when a client makes an objection to a price?
- Have we explained to our team the level of our costs in order to make them understand and share the need to defend our level of prices to ensure the business is sustainable?

GOOD PRACTICE 3

Definition of the practice's mission

- Have we succeeded in reflecting the mission of our practice in writing?
- Does it define precisely what our market is, who our customers are and what is expected of us?
- Does our team know it?
- Have we discussed it with them?
- Have we described where we would like to take our business in 15-20 years time?

The mission statement of a veterinary practice is developed by answering the following questions:

- **What is the purpose of my business?**
- **Who are my customers?**
- **What do the clients that I deal with really value?**
- **What must my business provide them with in order to satisfy them?**

Example of a mission statement*

"The mission of our veterinary practice is to provide those owners who enjoy a close, affectionate relationship with their pets with a comprehensive range of care, quality products and services that enable them to fully enjoy this relationship"

*(For a first opinion practice located in a suburb of a medium-sized city).

GOOD PRACTICE 4

Job descriptions

- Do we have written job descriptions for all the positions in our organisation?
- Do they include a list of duties and responsibilities, the organisational structure and evaluation criteria?
- Are we sure these descriptions are working documents that our employees know and use or that are updated regularly?

Job Description

Position: receptionist.

Responsible to: the manager of the veterinary practice.

General purpose and objective of post

To play an important role in the way that clients perceive the quality of services provided, whilst at reception or on the telephone.

To have responsibility for answering the telephone promptly and efficiently, arranging appointments with pet owners and maintaining a high standard of cleanliness and tidiness in the reception area. To have responsibility for managing key information to enable pet owners to know and understand the services offered by the practice.

To have an important role in the management of administrative services provided (estimates, invoicing and payments).

Main responsibilities

Administration

- Maximise the number of appointments, optimising the appointment book.
- Keep the information updated about the services provided by the practice and make it available to clients.
- Manage the system of booster and check-up reminders with clients.
- Keep client information constantly updated.

Finance

- Ensure that all services provided at the practice are invoiced and paid for.
- Minimize the number of unpaid accounts, promptly reporting them to management and following them up with clients.

Customer care

- Be attentive to pet owners who are waiting to be seen. Record and pass on messages.
- Keep the reception area neat, clean, well-ventilated and looking professional.
- Maintain a professional, kind and respectful attitude, both in person at reception and on the telephone.
- Record and pass on any complaints.
- Ensure that no clients leave the practice without either a new appointment scheduled or an updated appointment card.

Evaluation criteria

- Reception is always immaculate and organised.
- The appointment book is well managed.
- The telephone is well attended.
- Customer satisfaction (satisfaction surveys).
- Satisfaction from the rest of the team (vets and auxiliary staff).
- Percentage of boosters and clients retained.

GOOD PRACTICE **5**

Setting individual objectives for all employees of the practice, consistent with the mission and objectives of the practice

- Does each one of our employees have a number of objectives laid down in writing?
- Are they regularly updated?
- Are these objectives in accordance with the general objectives of the practice?
- Are these objectives ambitious but achievable, clear, within the area of responsibility of the employee and time-limited?

Individual Objectives

Position: receptionist.

Period: first quarter.

Objectives

- Increase the compliance rate for booster reminders from 72% to 75%.
- Ensure that at least 70% of clients leave with their next appointment already scheduled.
- Obtain an average rating of 8 (out of 10) on the question that relates to reception in the satisfaction surveys from new clients.
- Keep the number of debts below 1% of turnover.
- Update information on mobile phone numbers and email addresses for at least 75% of the clients seen during the period.
- Correctly manage the telephone switchboard changeover.

GOOD PRACTICE **6**

Regular staff performance appraisals

- Do we meet regularly with employees to monitor progress against objectives set?
- Do we analyse any variation and take mutually agreed corrective action?
- Do we link the results of these performance appraisals to the salary reviews or bonus schemes of our employees?

Performance Evaluation Programme					
Position: Receptionist/customer care			**Period under evaluation: (T1: First quarter)**		
Objective (Description)	**Measure (Objective specification)**	**Result obtained by the employee**	**Grade (Scale 0-12)**	**Relative relevance (% over 100)**	**Score**
1. Increase the percentage of boosters	Ensure booster rates go from 70% to 75%	Decreased to 66%	0	25%	0
2. Increase the client retention rate	Ensure that at least 70% of visitors attend the scheduled appointment (this measure is not available yet)	Reached 55%	6	20%	1.2
3. Client satisfaction with reception	Obtain an average rating of 8 (out of 10) on the question that relates to reception in the satisfaction surveys from new clients.	Rating of 8.5 from reception surveys taken	12	20%	2.4
4. Minimise debts, chase debtors	Keep the number of debts below 1% of turnover	It remained around 1%	10	15%	1.5
5. Improve the quality of the data in the client records	Obtain mobile phone numbers and email addresses for at least 75% of the pet owners that will visit us during the period	This data was obtained from 60% of pet owners visiting us	7	10%	0.7
6. Correctly manage calls on the switchboard	New switchboard to come into operation on 15th March, without disruption to service. Auxilary staff trained in its operation	The new switchboard started without serious problems on 10th March. The staff received training	9	10%	0.9
				Final Score	6.7

Summary of results and observations

Final score of the performance evaluation programme by objectives

In general, a satisfactory result. The most obvious area for improvement is the management of booster reminders.

Overlooked the follow-up calls for the overdue booster reminders sent by post, although there were some time constraints due to her having to temporarily replace another nurse who was off sick.

GOOD PRACTICE 7

Measuring employee productivity

- Do we measure the income generated by our vets?
- Do we have a clearly-defined system for recording the income generated by each vet for procedures involving several employees?
- Do we compare this income with the wage cost of each employee?
- Do we share the results of these productivity analyses with our employees?
- Do we link the results of these performance evaluations to the salary reviews or bonus schemes of our employees?

GOOD PRACTICE 8

Incentives for employees linked to customer satisfaction

- Do we have data relating to customer satisfaction that is objective and allows comparison between different periods?
- Do we inform our employees about the progress of this satisfaction data?
- Do we use this data as performance evaluation criteria for our employees?
- Do we link a variable part of our employees´ pay to these customer satisfaction results? (see questionnaire on the next page).

GOOD PRACTICE 9

Structured process for the recruitment and selection of new employees

- Do we have a formally-defined procedure for the recruitment and selection of new employees?
- Who in our organisation takes part in this process?
- Do we use any outside help?
- What kind of selection procedure do we use?
- Do we have a defined format for the the interviews?
- Have we defined the training and induction programme for a new employee?

Questionnaire to measure customer satisfaction

The quality of the service we offer is very important to us.

Please set aside 3 minutes of your time to answer these questions.

Please circle the number that best describes the experience you have had with us today	**Very poor**	**Poor**	**Good**	**Excellent**
A. Telephone Service				
1. Rapid response to your call	1	2	3	4
2. Courteous and efficient receptionist	1	2	3	4
3. Your questions were answered clearly	1	2	3	4
B. Our Reception				
1. Our staff were friendly and efficient	1	2	3	4
2. Your waiting time was reasonable	1	2	3	4
3. Your questions were answered clearly	1	2	3	4
4. You were comfortable and well looked after while you were waiting	1	2	3	4
C. Our Facilities				
1. It was easy to get here	1	2	3	4
2. The entrance was well signposted	1	2	3	4
3. The hospital was very clean	1	2	3	4
4. There were no bad odors	1	2	3	4
5. There was interesting reading material in reception	1	2	3	4
D. The Consulting Room				
1. The professionalism of our nurses	1	2	3	4
2. The nurses were helpful	1	2	3	4
3. You were comfortable while your pet was being examined	1	2	3	4
4. Cleanliness and tidiness of the consulting room	1	2	3	4
E. Our Vets				
1. The vet gave you enough time	1	2	3	4
2. The vet explained everything that they were doing well	1	2	3	4
3. Your questions were well answered	1	2	3	4
4. How thorough was the physical examination of your pet?	1	2	3	4
How would you rate our overall service?	1	2	3	4
The next time you have to go to the vet, do you think you will return to our practice?		Yes	No	

GOOD PRACTICE **10**

Existence of programmes to promote staff retention

- Have we defined a typical career path for our employees?
- Have we defined a series of salary increments and non-financial benefits (working hours) for our good employees to improve their position over time?
- Do we try to promote their professional development within our organisation?

GOOD PRACTICE **11**

Measuring employee satisfaction

- Do we regularly and objectively measure the level of employee satisfaction?
- Do we try to detect areas of dissatisfaction?
- Do we analyse the dynamics of cooperation or competition that exist between the different groups in our team?
- Do we regularly hold some kind of meeting with the aim of sharing and disseminating information as well as being a way to improve the coordination between all our employees?

GOOD PRACTICE **12**

Measuring the net flow of patients at the practice

- Do we know how many new patients joined last year?
- Do we know how many patient deaths there were?
- Do we know how many patients have stopped coming?
- Do we know how many former patients have been recovered?

Flow of patients in a veterinary practice

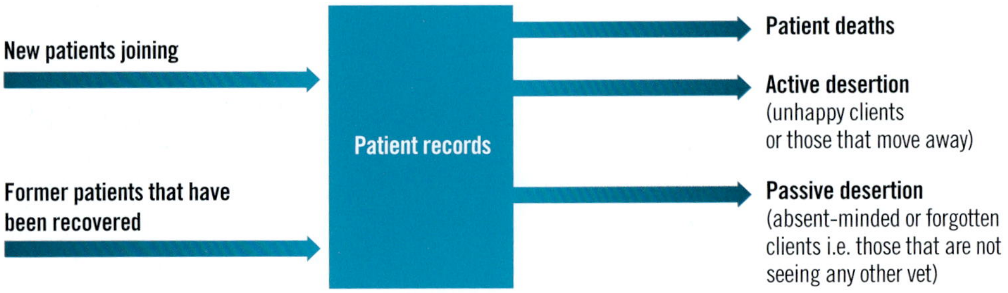

GOOD PRACTICE **13**

Measuring loyalty and programmes for the recovery of lost clients

- Do we quantify the clients that are lost over the course of a year?
- Do we make any methodical, systematic and organised effort to find out the causes behind these client and patient losses and recover them?

GOOD PRACTICE **14**

Measuring the economic value of a patient to the business

- Do we ever calculate the average life span of a patient for our business?
- Do we ever calculate the economic value of a patient to our business over the course of that average life span?

GOOD PRACTICE **15**

Newsletters or news bulletins

- Do we use newsletters or some other form of regular communication with our clients in order to keep them informed of our services, matters of general interest for pet owners, etc?

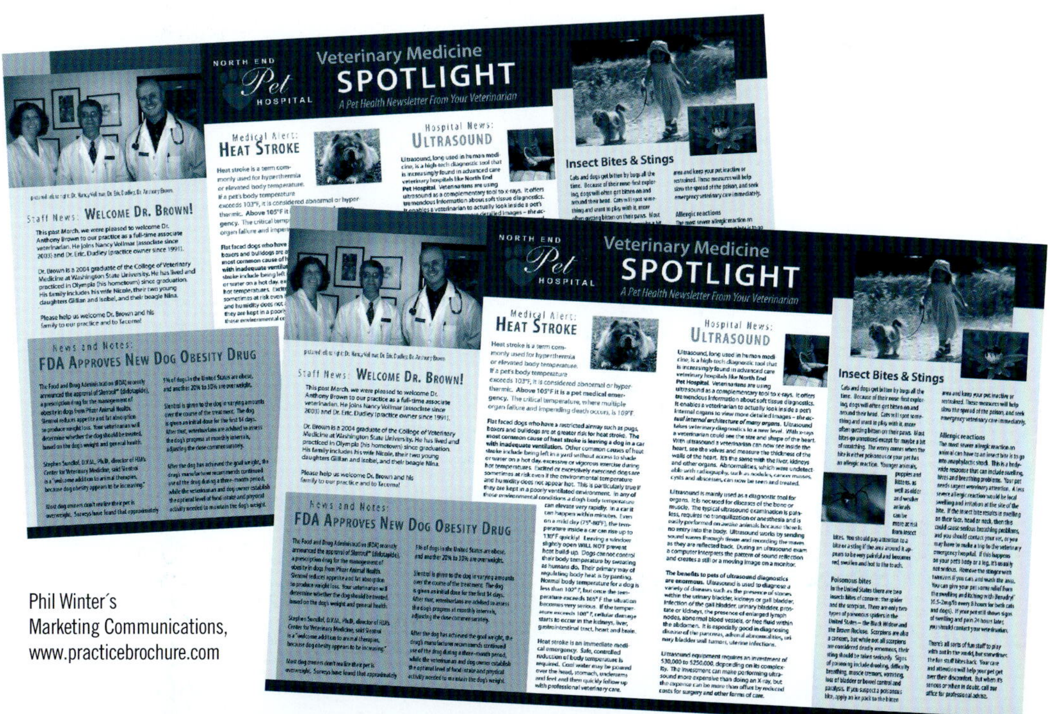

North End Pet Hospital
Veterinary Medicine SPOTLIGHT
A Pet Health Newsletter From Your Veterinarian
Medical Alert: Heat Stroke
Hospital News: Ultrasound
Insect Bites & Stings
Staff News: Welcome Dr. Brown!
News and Notes: FDA Approves New Dog Obesity Drug

Phil Winter´s Marketing Communications, www.practicebrochure.com

GOOD PRACTICE **16**

Up-to-date information about our services

- Do we have up-to-date, written information (in the form of a leaflet or similar) that is readily available to our clients?
- Are there any notice or information boards at reception indicating the services provided?
- Are there photographs of facilities or equipment that cannot be seen from reception?

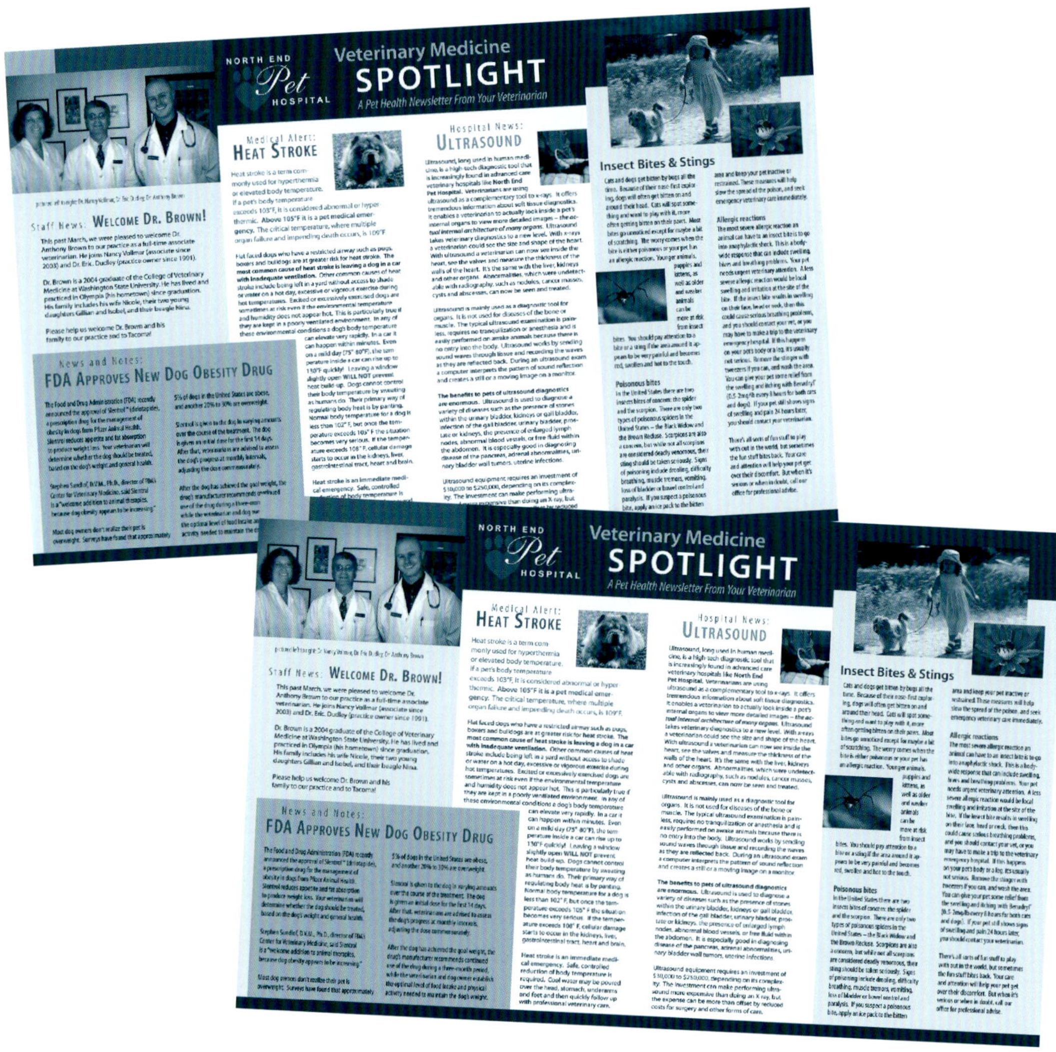

Phil Winter´s
Marketing Communications,
www.practicebrochure.com

GOOD PRACTICE **17**

Open channels to listen to "the voice of the client"

- Do we talk to our clients about the quality of service that we provide?
- Do we ask them for improvement suggestions in an organised way?
- Do we occasionally hold focus groups with them?
- Do we have a system that is flexible, reliable and convenient for the client that enables us to gather service complaints?

GOOD PRACTICE **18**

Promote and encourage client recommendation

- Do we encourage our clients to recommend us to their friends and acquaintances?
- Have we ever openly told them that we like them recommending us?
- Do we make the job of recommending us easy by giving them some kind of written information?
- Do we reward or thank them for the people they have sent us?

GOOD PRACTICE **19**

Telephone service standards

- Do we control the quality of our telephone service?
- Have we defined call standards (within how many rings a call will be answered, which telephone greeting is used, how to answer standard questions, which calls must be made proactively, by whom and how calls are returned)?

GOOD PRACTICE **20**

Customer care for new clients

- Do we write a welcome letter to all our new clients within 24 hours of them coming to our practice?
- Do we send them a leaflet with a description of our services?
- Do we ask for their opinion on the service they received on the day they first used our service?

The reader will have realised that several of these good practice points are interrelated. In fact, some of them refer to the management of human resources (the employees), others to the financial control of the business and so on. The following classification groups and reorders the twenty good practice points by **management area.**

Good business management practices

Good practice - description	Management area
Definition of the practice's mission statement	Business vision
Setting individual objectives for employees consistent with the mission and objectives of the practice	
There are incentives linked to customer satisfaction for employees	
Measurement of employee productivity (individually and collectively)	
Regular review and interpretation of the practice's financial results	Financial control
A well-defined pricing policy	
Regular staff performance appraisals, both verbally and in writing	Staff development
Written job descriptions for all employees	
Measurement of employee satisfaction	
Structured process for the recruitment and selection of new employees	
Existence of programmes and plans to promote staff retention	
To measure the degree of client loyalty and have recovery programmes for lost clients	Client loyalty
Encourage and reward those clients that recommend our practice to other potential clients	
Measure the net flow of patients over a period of time	Client retention
Open channels to listen to the voice of the client (focus groups, solicit improvement suggestions)	
Calculate the "value of a client" to the business over the period of their life span.	
Use newsletters or other regular forms of written communication with clients	
Customer care for new clients: send a welcome and thank you letter	
Have a current leaflet with a detailed description of the practice's services	
Telephone service standards: defined protocols, do regular quality checks	

A call for optimism

We should neither be too surprised or disheartened if the number of these good practice points currently in use in our veterinary practice is small. Both in the United States as in Spain and Portugal[4], it is a minority of vets that consistently apply these good management practices.

Use of good management practices in different countries

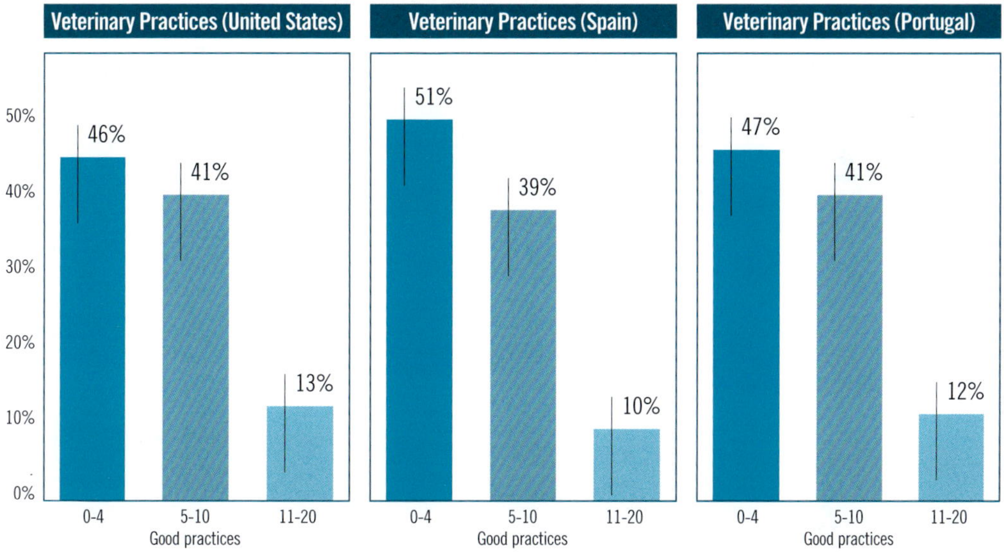

The optimistic interpretation of this scenario is that there is considerable scope for improvement in business performance in our veterinary practices. The gradual inclusion of these good management practices will become even more relevant in markets with a highly competitive environment, and obviously essential in the case of practices and organisations that aspire to grow in the next few years.

This is not about being weighed down or paralysed by the prospect of an unachievable task, but rather to objectively assess where one stands and to set some objectives for gradual improvement. The rest of this manual tries to pave the way for the manager to implement these principles in their veterinary practice in a practical way.

Key Chapter Concepts

- The business performance of a veterinary practice is not a matter of chance or luck.
- There are some well-known factors that affect its results, some of which are controllable by the vet.
- The systematic use of good business management practices improves the probability of business success. Most vets do not make enough use of these practices.
- In a competitive market environment, the veterinary practices that want to grow will have to gradually implement these practices.

References

1. Volk, J. Executive summary of the AVMA-Pfizer business practices study. JAVMA, Vol 226, No.2, Jan 15, 2005, pp. 212-218.
2. AVEPA - Hill's Pet Nutrition. Estudio de Cumplimiento, 2006.
3. Hellriegel, D. Management, 8th edition, Cincinnati, OH, South-Western Publishing Co., 1999, 4-36, pp. 355-378.
4. Author´s own work based on surveys of veterinary practice owners who attended management courses taught by the author.

The management
of the veterinary practice

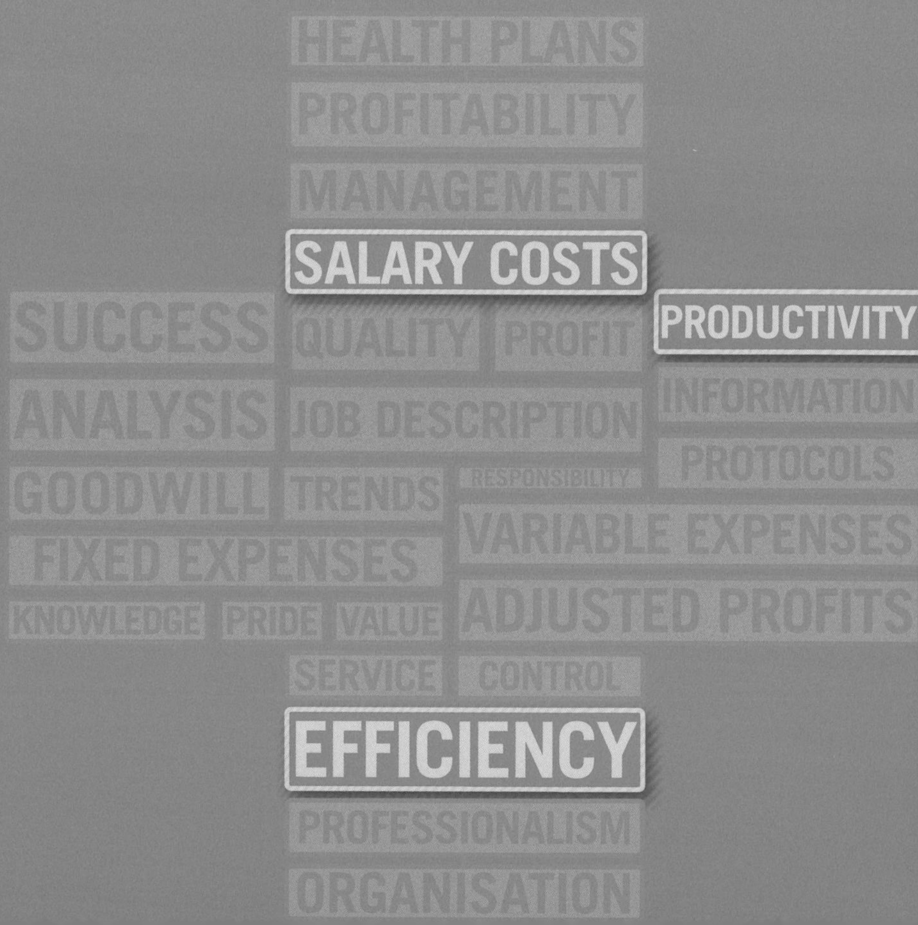

2

Is it really necessary to manage?

Many veterinary practices are small or medium-sized businesses that cannot afford to take on highly-qualified professional managers. The management of these businesses is not a simple task however; you have to motivate and supervise a team of personnel, you have to offer a quality service to customers, you have to communicate effectively both internally and externally, you have to have good inventory control... The list is endless and, on occasions, overwhelming. Just to make things even more difficult, the vast majority of the owners of these practices never received any management training whilst studying to become a vet. What is more, their vocation is not to manage a business, but to practice veterinary medicine. In other words, many vets get into management more out of obligation than conviction.

When someone goes from being **an employed vet to becoming the owner of a veterinary practice**, a major change takes place with implications that many are reluctant to accept. While the employed vet focuses on meeting the needs of patients and their owners, the obligations of the owner of a **veterinary business** go well beyond that point. The business owner has additional ethical, legal and professional responsibilities: to the other partners (if there are any), commercial suppliers, the state and to their employees. In many large businesses, the ownership and management of the business are separated. The owner of a veterinary practice is not obliged to also be the manager but they are required to ensure that **someone** manages the business. The different models and solutions to the issue of managing a practice will be addressed in the remainder of this chapter.

The difference between being a vet and managing a veterinary practice

What is the mission of the Principal of a veterinary practice?

While the effectiveness of a vet can be measured by what they **do**, the effectiveness of the veterinary practice Principal is measured by what they **make others do**. A good Principal or manager must plan, organise, lead and supervise the use of human and material resources at their veterinary practice to enable it to achieve its objectives.

This means that they must spend time and be committed to lead their team. According to Caroline Jevring[1], the Principal of a veterinary practice must divide their time roughly as follows:

- Administrative tasks <10%.
- Commercial management <10%.
- Customer relations <20%.
- Clinical work <20%.

Training, motivating, monitoring and evaluating the team (vets and non-vets) would take **the remainder of the time, up to 60%.**

If the owner of the veterinary practice is not able, or lacks the necessary motivation, to devote a significant proportion of their time to people management, then their obligation as owner is to delegate this responsibility to a professional manager.

Managerial tasks

Is it really necessary to have a manager in a veterinary practice? What are the tasks that a person in this role has to undertake?

Figure 1 shows the managerial tasks for a veterinary practice. This list has been adapted from the original by Shilcock[2].

Figure 1. Managerial Tasks at the Veterinary Practice.

Personnel Management
Selection and recruitment
Job descriptions
Contracts
Induction training
Continuous Professional Development
Payroll
Determine salary bands
Performance appraisals
Rota – timetables
Data Management
Software updates
Hardware updates
Management Reports
Training
Financial Management
Accounting
Bank relations
Cash flow (treasury) management
Stock control
Purchases
Debt Control
Insurance
Financial Planning
Management of marketing and services
Pricing policy
Development new services
Promotion of the practice
Communication with clients
Advertising and publications
Meetings - events at the practice
Marketing planning
General Administration
General purchases
Investments
Creation of protocols
Complaints management
Internal communication
Practice Manual

Here it is possible to appreciate the wide variety of tasks that need to be undertaken beyond that of practicing veterinary medicine. The tasks are grouped into thematic areas: personnel management, management of information systems, financial management, marketing and services management and general information. Within each of these areas are different tasks.

These tasks can be carried out by a managing partner (i.e. the owner or one of the owners of the practice) or by a professional manager. A couple of points need to be clarified however. Some of these tasks that are considered to be of strategic importance (like for example the selection and recruitment of personnel, determining salary bands or the pricing policy) should be approved by the owner or owners of the practice, whether or not they were originally designed and proposed by a professional manager. Other tasks, of a more tactical or technical nature (like for example the accounting, stock control, or communication policy with clients), can be almost entirely delegated to a professional manager.

Practical solutions: Who should be the manager?

A similar development takes place in many veterinary practices with regard to management tasks:

- At first, it is the owner (or one of the partners) who starts spending a few hours a week on managerial tasks. Sometimes, if there is more than one partner, they do it on a rotational basis regardless of their individual capabilities or interests.

- As the practice grows, things get more complex and the managerial tasks need ever more time and skills. This forces the owner to start spending at least half of their time on management issues. This is accompanied by a period of transition and uncertainty, in which the owner starts for the first time to seriously consider employing a professional manager. The main obstacles to taking this decision include the fear of losing control of the business, the difficulty in finding a person with the right profile and concern at the financial burden that hiring a qualified professional will entail for the business (particularly as that professional is seemingly "non productive", i.e. not doing consultations with clients).

- When the veterinary center exceeds a certain size, the decision to appoint a dedicated manager is inevitable. Sometimes it is the same owner who decides to "hang up his hat" for good and focus on the management of their practice. On other occasions they opt for employing a professional manager (sometimes part-time to start with).

Financial analysis conducted in American clinics estimates that a veterinary practice can spend between 3% and 5% of its annual revenue on paying someone to manage a practice. If we also take this rule as being good for practices in other countries, this will provide us with a theoretical indicator for practices of different sizes to budget for in this department.

Figure 2. How much can be allocated to recruiting a professional manager.

Annual turnover		Allocation
Less than 400,000 monetary units annual turnover	→	It is hardly possible to recruit anyone to help with these tasks.
Between 400,000 and 600,000 monetary units annual turnover	→	Some 20,000 monetary units annual gross
From 600,000 monetary units to 1,000,000 monetary units of annual turnover	→	Some 30,000 monetary units annual gross
From 1,000,000 to 2,000,000 monetary units annually	→	Up to 75,000 monetary units annual gross

These bands will establish the profile of the professional that we can aim to recruit. In the first and second salary bands, we would normally have access to recent graduates or young professionals. The third band will enable us to recruit an experienced professional.

A variety of profiles can work equally well when developing a management role at a veterinary practice:

- In the absence of specific higher qualifications in the sector (in most countries there are no university programmes for training veterinary managers, with some rare exceptions), an alternative solution could be to recruit a graduate in Business Administration and Management. They can be trained up in the veterinary practice under the tutelage of the owners.

- Another option to consider might be to recruit someone part-time who has business training and wider management experience but for personal reasons prefers to work part-time.

- Another alternative would be the internal promotion of someone on the team. A competent receptionist or a head nurse with the necessary attitude and capabilities can become a good manager, especially if we invest in their training.

- Finally, there is always the option of the owner (or one of the partners) deciding to swap the stethoscope for the calculator in order to take on the management tasks for their practice. In this scenario it is also recommended that this person supplements their academic veterinary training with a professional development programme in management. Before taking this decision, it would be a good idea to assess the loss of income that this owner could have produced as a vet. According to a shocking study conducted in the United States for NCVEI (National Commission of Veterinary Economic Issues)[3], the profitability of many veterinary practices was negatively affected when the owner reduced their clinical work in favour of management. The best results are seen when a non-veterinary professional is put in charge of management.

Key management indicators: What information can be analysed at a veterinary practice

In most veterinary practices there is more information than can be analysed for practical purposes. In fact, more than **information**, there is just **data** (information that has not been processed and is waiting to be interpreted). Management programmes used by practices contain thousands of entries with data on transactions, clients, medical procedures, etc. More than one vet has been disappointed after spending all morning delving into data listings in the search for answers, to end up more lost that they were at the start of the session...

Management literature[4] has popularised the term KPI (Key Performance Indicators) to refer to the **key management indicators of a business**. This is a limited range of quantitative measures that summarise the maximum amount of relevant information in the least possible space. The particular range of KPIs to monitor depends on the core business model of the practice and the priorities defined by both owner and management.

The model in **figure 3**[5] describes the logical relationships that exisit between income, expenditure and the profitability of the veterinary practice, suggesting a wide range of indicators.

Figure 3. Profitability model of a Veterinary Practice.

Annual income = the number of active patient records x average annual visits x average revenue per visit		
Objective 1	**Objective 2**	**Objective 3**
Increase the number of active patient records	**Increase the average number of annual visits per patient**	**Increase the average income per visit**
Indicators	Indicators	Indicators
1. Death rate of patients. 2. Drop-out rate of patients. 3. Number of new patients. 4. Number of patients that have been recovered.	5. Average annual visits per patient. 6. % of active patient records without any "R"s. 7. % of active patient records without reminders. 8. % of active patient records without scheduled appointments.	9. Average income per visit. 10. Number of items per invoice. 11. % of active patient records with transactions in the surgery and in the shop. 12. Diagnostic ratio (diagnostic tests/ medical services).

Annual profitability = annual income – annual expenses
Objective 4: efficiency, productivity, control of expenses
Indicators
13. Salary cost (all staff) as % of turnover for the period. 14. Productivity of each vet (income from medical services from each vet/ their total salary cost to the business). 15. Purchase cost of "consumables" not chargeable as a % of the income from medical services. 16. Purchase cost of "chargeable items" as % of revenue generate by the shop.

The income of a veterinary practice is the result of three factors: the number of patients, the frequency with which they come and the average spend on each visit. Indicators 1 to 12 aim to measure these variables:

1. **Annual death rate of patients (as %).** This is calculated by dividing the number of animals that died over the course of a year by the number of active patient records that the practice had at the beginning of that same year and then multiplying the result by one hundred. It should be remembered that what we understand to be an active patient is one that has made at least one transaction with the practice in the last 12 months.

2. **The annual drop-out rate of patients (as %).** To calculate this, we first have to find out how many patients have "abandoned" our practice in the past 12 months. For that we need to count those patients that made at least one financial transaction with the practice in the period between the last 24 and 12 months but have not made any transactions in the last 12 months. Once we have calculated the number of patients that have dropped-out, we divide that figure by the number of active patient records at the start of the year and multiply it by one hundred.

3. **Number of new patients (as %).** For this we calculate the number of patients that have made a financial transaction in our practice for the first time in the last 12 months, divide this by the number of active patient records at the start of the period and multipy this by one hundred. For the purposes of this analysis, it would be advisable to separate referred patients and emergencies as their special nature prevents them from being considered "regular patients" at our practice.

4. **Number of patients "recovered" (as %).** This refers to those patients that had abandoned the practice in the previous few years and that more recently have returned, making at least one financial transaction.

Note: The net flow of clients throughout the year will result from the combination of the four previous indicators, as per the following equation:

Number of active patient records
at the start of the year
- Patient deaths
+ New patients
- Lost patients
+ Recovered patients

= The number of active patients at the end of the year

In fact, it is not uncommon to find veterinary practices that lose between 30 and 50% of their clients every year (counting deaths and those that drop-out...). In a market environment in which pet ownership is not expected to increase, this data is worrying and merits close monitoring by veterinary practice managers. Many (the majority) of these desertions are not due to customer dissatisfaction, but simply because they forgot or their vets failed to communicate with them.

5. **Average annual visits per patient**. This is calculated by dividing the total number of "visits" (=transactions) made by patients throughout the year by the number of active patients. An improvement on this indicator would be to distinguish between "surgery" visits and "shop" visits and to calculate the annual average for both.

6. **Average active patient records without any "R"s**. This indicator refers to the famous programme of the 3 Rs (re-call, re-check, reminder) popularised by T. Catanzaro[6]. This consists in calculating what percentage of the active patient records do not have a note on their medical record of any future scheduled appointment, no overdue reminders and no telephone call to be made. This is an indicator of the future rate of lost clients, as these are patients that will only return to the practice if the owner takes the initiative.

7. **Average active patient records without reminders.** This refers only to the percentage of our active records that do not have any reminders for future treatment in our practice flagged up.

8. **Average active records without a scheduled appointment**. This refers to the percentage of our active records that do not have a future appointment scheduled with the practice. Well-planned preventative medicine and appropriate client monitoring are a must if we want to improve the frequency rates of client visits. If we really want to see our clients more often, it should be us that "pulls our weight" rather than leave the initiative to the client.

9. **Average transaction fee.** This is calculated by dividing the practice's annual income by the total number of visits (or transactions). An improvement on this measure would consist in calculating the average income per "clinical" visit and the average income per "shop" visit. Some authors[7] consider that the "clinical" average transaction fee should be around three times the cost of a first consultation at the practice.

10. **Number of items (or services) per invoice.** This indicator reflects the extent to which clients that come to our practice use just one or more of our services and/or products.

11. **Percentage of active records with transactions in the shop and in the surgery.** This tells us the extent to which we have been successful at making "cross sales" between our medical services and the products in our shop.

12. **Diagnostic ratio.** This is calculated as the % that represents income from diagnostic tests over the total income generated from medical services throughout the period. Some authors[8] estimate it at around 20%. Much higher figures would indicate abuse or inefficiency in performing diagnostic tests whilst much lower figures would indicate inadequate medical protocols or insufficient diagnostic equipment at the practice.

    At this point, it would be a good idea to analyse the main cost centres for the practice as their ultimate profitability will depend on their size in proportion to turnover. Indicators 13 to 16 aim to measure these costs and the variables that affect them:

13. **Total salary cost of staff as a percentage of the turnover of the practice**. The wage cost is the largest cost centre on the management accounts of a veterinary practice. This indicator has a key impact on the profitability of the centre. In general, it is considered difficult for the practice to achieve reasonable profits if it allocates much more than 40% of its income to cover salary costs (and in particular more than 20-25% to cover the costs of veterinary salaries).

14. **The productivity of each vet.** This refers to income generated by each vet from clinical services, divided by the salary cost of that vet to the business. It enables us to assess the past performance of each vet and identify relevant differences within our team. We must remember that elements such as experience, hours worked, clinical specialty and the number and level of training of nurses will all have an important influence on the values of this particular indicator.

15. **The cost of non-chargeable consumables.** This is the expenditure on clinical supplies that are not chargeable as a percentage of the turnover from clinical services. It gives us guidance on the efficiency and judicious use of resources by our team.

16. **The cost of chargeable items.** These include both drug and shop stock purchases, as a percentage of turnover from the sale of shop stock and drugs. This indicator enables us to calculate the profit margin on these product lines as well as helping us to identify possible inefficiencies in stock management.

A good management software programme should, in a relatively automated way, allow for the collection, trend identification and interpretation of these indicators... The real "art" of a good manager resides in implementing the measures (plans, programmes, concrete actions) required to return those indicators with negative deviations back to the "area of normality".

As business managers, we should not settle for knowing that "this year I have grown 12%". Do we know how we have achieved this 12%? What has been our net flow of active patients? How many lost clients have we had? Are clients coming to our practice with more or less frequency? Which kind of visits are they coming for: the shop or the surgery? What is the average transaction fee per visit for the shop and the surgery? etc... The control of these key variables, and their regular analysis, will enable us to take better control of our business and to implement the most appropriate actions for each situation.

Management report: Summarising key information to make decisions

At this point, more than one reader may feel overwhelmed at the magnitude of the task ahead: where to begin?

A very useful tool in medium and large businesses is the management report. This consists of condensing the most relevant information relating to the running of the business in a given period into a single document. As the reader will have already guessed, the management report amounts to a concise and organised list of KPIs (key performance indicators), accompanied by their corresponding interpretation.

This report is always prepared on the same dates (for example on the last week of the month or quarter) and is always presented to the owners on the same dates (for example the first non-bank holiday Monday of the month or the first non-bank holiday Monday of the quarter).

In large organisations, a fixed format tends to be established for this report in order to make collection of the necessary data more systematic. It also facilitates comparison between periods and makes interpretation a part of the management report. If properly drafted, this report should enable the practice owners to have an accurate and detailed overview of what is happening, even if they are not physically present at the practice.

John Sheridan[9] proposes a check-list with the most relevant questions that a good management report should provide answers for. Figure 4 demonstrates this format:

Figure 4. Management Report.

Some general questions

- What was the turnover compared to that of the previous month? What was the turnover compared to the same month last year? What is this year's turnover to date?
- How many transactions took place this month compared to last month? How many transactions took place in the same month last year?
- Why were they higher (or lower)?
- What was the distribution of income between clinical services and product sales?
- What was the distribution of income per vet and per type of clinical service?
- What has been the best thing that has happened this month?
- What has been the worst thing that has happened this month?
- What have we done about both things?

Some questions about the practice team

- Who has been on holiday, sick leave or travelling?
- What has the staff turnover been so far this year and how does it compare with the last year?
- What has been the total salary cost for all vets (owner(s) included) in comparison to the budget and with the previous year?
- What has been the wage cost of all non-veterinary staff in comparison with the budget and with the previous year?
- What has been the variation and how can it be explained?
- Have we measured the productivity of the veterinary team (income generated against salary costs) both collectively for the whole team and individually for each person?
- What have been the results of this analysis?
- Have we taken any action in response to these results?
- Have you received copies of the clinical reports prepared by the vets?
- How many times have we congratulated an employee this month? What has been the reason? Have we shared this with the rest of the team?

Some questions about the clients and the patients

- How many active patients do we have on our database? How does this figure compare with the previous month?
- How many new patients have come to the practice?
- How many patients have "deserted" (are no longer active) in the last month?
- What has been the average amount per transaction?
- What is the average spend per customer so far this year?
- How many clients at the "average spend per client" do we need to meet the practice's financial objectives?
- How many complaints have been registered this month?
- Which have been the three most serious ones?
- How many letters have we written and/or calls of thanks or congratulations have we made to our clients?

Some questions about drugs and consumables

- How much have we spent on drugs and consumables this month?
- What is the percentage of the amount spent on drugs and consumables with respect to the total income?
- What has been the variation with respect to that budgeted for?
- Why has this (positive or negative) variation occurred?
- What remedial action (if necessary) has been taken?
- When did we do the last physical stock check?
- What did we find?
- Have we had any significant issues with any of our suppliers?
- Have there been any signs of wastage, loss or theft of stock?

Some questions about the operation of the practice

- Do all our employees know how much we have to generate daily in order to be economically viable?
- What is the value of the unpaid invoices to date?
- What was the proportion of appointments available that were taken this month?
- How many hospitalisation kennels were occupied?
- What was the variation regarding the budget?
- Has there been any accident?
- Have there been any incidents related to health and safety?

Some questions about finance

- What has been the margin left by clinical services during the month? What has been the variation with respect to the budget?
- What has been the margin left by product sales during the month? What has been the variation with respect to the budget?
- What has our bank balance been at the end of the month?
- Have we been overdrawn? Is there a foreseeable risk of being overdrawn in the short term?

To conclude: some basic ideas regarding people management

It is no use controlling the figures and interpreting them if we forget the people behind them. In fact, data is the result of the peoples´ behaviour. They are not an objective in themselves, but a means to better understand what is happening.

Thus you should remember a series of basic rules that successful managers tend to respect when dealing with people:

1. Praise in public, criticism in private

We must always correct any unsatisfactory behaviour in our employees in private. Few things demotivate and cause more resentment in a professional than to be reprimanded before a client or colleagues. On the other hand we must take the opportunity to publically acknowledge the achievements and appropriate behaviour of our team. This reinforces the self-esteem of our team and will cement our leadership.

2. Information is power

It is not a good idea to reward or punish the team with information. Favoritism towards team members is perceived as a discriminatory comparison and is a common source of grievance. The employees of the veterinary practice closely observe the behaviour of the owner and take great note of any signs regarding possible preferences within the team. The way in which information is shared is also a powerful indicator of these preferences. For this reason, the owner must be particularly scrupulous when delivering information relevant to their team: news, investments, rolling out of new services, changes in wage policies, etc. Any important information should be delivered directly by the practice management to all those affected. This has the twin objective of controlling the message and showing that there are no preferences when communications are given. In this respect internal planning meetings are especially important.

3. Each person where they contribute the most

It is often said that the well-managed business is one where each task is assigned to the person on the team with the lowest salary and that ethically, legally and professionally can carry it out correctly. In other words, why have vets answering the telephone, checking temperatures, waiting for lab test results or taking blood samples, when well-trained support staff can carry out these tasks at a lower cost?

The real added value of a vet is in diagnosing, deciding and proposing treatments as well as performing complex medical procedures such as surgery. The veterinary practice that keeps their vets busy with these tasks will get the best performance.

4. Do not criticise colleagues, clients or former employees in front of the team

Doing this says nothing good about us, and warns our employees about what to expect the day they no longer work for us… If any of our employees display this behaviour, we should reprimand them politely but firmly.

5. Leading by example

Although we are not often aware of it, our employees closely observe the behaviour of the practice owner and tend to mimic it. Imitation has always been one of the most powerful ways that humans learn. The personality, style and work ethic of the owner permeates just about everything in the organisation, giving shape to the famous "corporate culture". Therefore, we should not ask our employees to do one thing whilst we daily demonstrate the opposite.

6. It is better to do a few things well rather than a lot of things badly…

One of the things that really undermines the credibility of a manager in front of their team is the bad habit of starting too many projects and hardly finishing any. It is better to focus on two, or at most three, important issues each year and complete them. The manager should prepare projects well, plan them, involve the team, monitor performance, take remedial action, re-involve the team, etc. If every time we read an article or attend a management course we return to the surgery with a brilliant idea then call together the team in order to convince them of the enormous importance of putting it into practice, then only a few weeks later forget to follow it up… What is the message we are sending to our team? What will happen the next time we try to embark on a project?

7. Be generous with the ownership of good ideas

The best managers are not those that take the credit for everything that happens. They are those that manage to get the best out of their team. Being able to get the team to "generate" good ideas is far more effective, motivating and positive for the working environment than to have to be always dictating what to do. Actually, sometimes the best ideas come spontaneously from someone in our team, in which case it is essential that we have the necessary wisdom and humility to acknowledge it before the rest of the team. On many other occasions however our challenge as managers will be to stimulate and guide the team so it is them that generates those good ideas. If we do this with enough skill and subtlety, we will manage to get them to adopt and support ideas that they perceive to be their own. After all, what matters is not from whom the idea originated but putting it into practice...

Key Chapter Concepts

- Spending many hours working in the practice does not mean you are managing it. Managerial tasks require dedication and specific skills. If the owner of the practice is unwilling or unable to manage, they are obliged to employ someone to do it.

- There are several ways to manage the practice: giving the responsibility part or full-time to one of the partners, internally promoting someone who can be trusted or employing an outside professional. The best solution will depend on the size of the practice and its stage of development.

- It is important to learn to select and analyse the most relevant information. The key performance indicators and management reports are two tools that, if properly used, will help the veterinary practice to better control their financial health.

- It is not data but people who are responsible for the success of the business. There are some basic rules that we must both understand and respect if we want to successfully lead a team.

References

1. Jevring, C. *Managing a Veterinary Practice*, 2nd ed. Saunders Elsevier, 2007.
2. Shilcock, M. *et al. Veterinary Practice Management, A Practical Guide*. Saunders, 2003.
3. Wasserman, N. What is the Most Efficient Way for Veterinarians to Manage Their Practice? NCVEI (www.ncvei.org).
4. Kaplan, R. et al. Balanced Scored Card: Translating Strategy into Action. Harvard Business School Press, 1996.
5. First published in the journal Argos Nº 90 (July/August 2007).
6. Catanzaro, T. *et al.* Veterinary Healthcare Services, Options in Delivery. Iowa State University Press, 2000.
7. Well Managed Practices Study (www.wellmp.com)
8. Moreau, P. Practice Financial Indicators: Measure Your Productivity. EJCAP, October 2005, Vol. 15, Issue 2.
9. www.veterinarybusinessbriefing.com

The profitability of the veterinary practice:
How to measure it and what it depends on

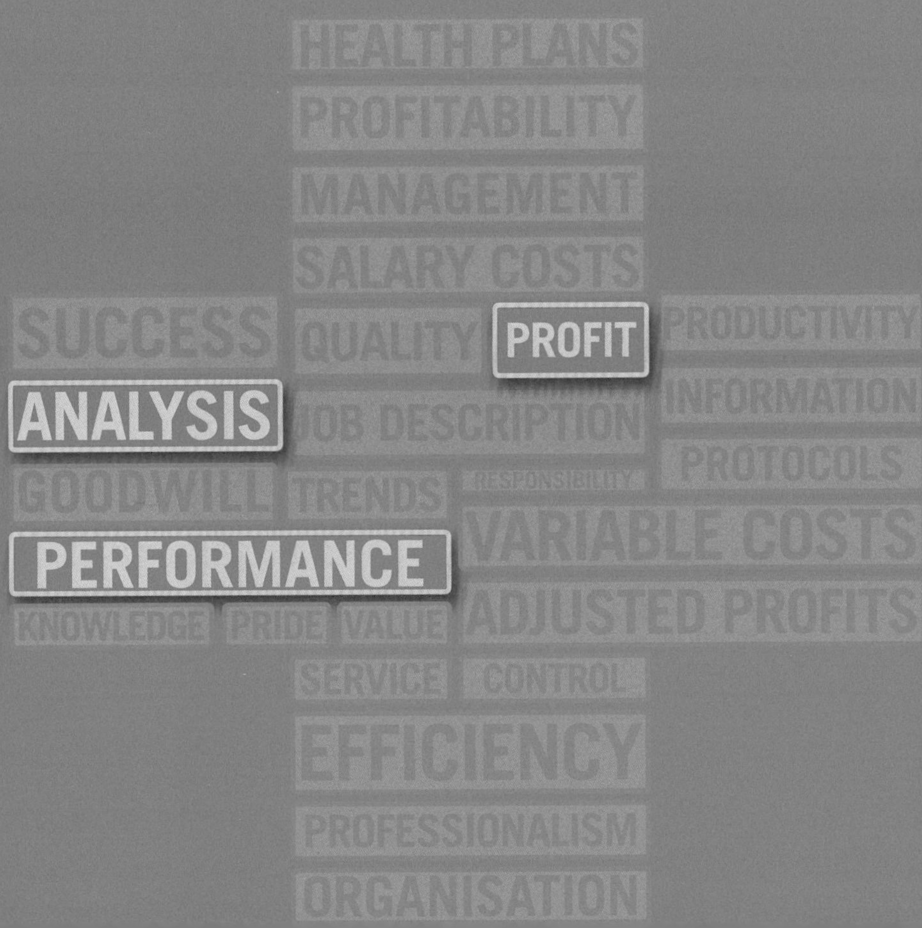

3

The profitability of a veterinary practice is the result of the evolution of income and expenditure incurred over a fixed period of time. The difference between the income and expenditure in each period will provide us with an **absolute measure** of profitability: **profit** (in monetary units).

Profit for a given period

=

Income for that period – expenses from that period

A common method of assessing whether this net profit (in monetary units) is high or low is to compare it with other figures such as, for example, total practice income in the same period. In this way, we get a **relative measure** of profitability known as a **profit margin** which is calculated as a percentage.

Profit margin (%)

=

$$\frac{\text{Practice profits over a given period x 100}}{\text{Practice income for that period}}$$

Another interesting option could be to compare the net profit for the period with investment in net assets (value net of debts) that the owner or owners of the practice have made in their business. There are several variants of this calculation although perhaps ROA or **return on net assets** is one of the most common.

ROA (return on net assets, %)

=

$$\frac{\text{Profits from the practice in the period x 100}}{\text{Net Value of business assets}}$$

The usefulness of ROA lies in the fact that we can assess to what degree this business is efficiently using its resources in order to generate proportionally acceptable profits.

Analysis of practice income

Information about the income generated from a veterinary practice can be presented in various formats, depending on the type of analysis that you want to undertake.

This author proposes to use the following information structure that allows you to distinguish between the main sources of income that are most commonly seen in a veterinary practice.

Figure 1. Sources of income.

Breakdown of income from a veterinary practice (fictitious data)	Monetary Units
Revenue from consultations	51,966
Revenue from vaccinations	46,621
Revenue from microchips	8,909
Revenue from wormers and flea control	7,424
Revenue from surgery	56,718
Revenue from hospitalisations	22,568
Revenue from diagnostic imaging (X-rays, ultrasonography...)	24,944
Revenue from blood tests	43,058
Revenue from emergencies	30,289
Revenue from home visits	4,454
Total for the surgery (clinical services)	**296,951**
Revenue from drugs	74,148
Revenue from pet food (prescription diets and life-stage)	21,711
Revenue from pet accessories	10,105
Revenue from shampoos and hygiene products	8,175
Revenue from grooming (if applicable)	13,126
Total for shop and other services	**127,265**
Total revenue for the veterinary practice	**424,216**

Once we have this information available, we can make three kinds of interesting analyses.

1. Relative importance of each income source

This consists in calculating what percentage each source of income represents against the total revenue of the practice. This analysis will allow us to quantify to what level our veterinary practice depends on, or is focused on, a particular type of activity. It also enables us to detect important differences with other veterinary practices, which can be a sign that one source of income is either under or well-developed in our practice.

Figure 2. Value of the different lines of income shown as a percentage.

Breakdown of income from a veterinary practice (fictitious data)	Monetary Units	% of total income
Revenue from consultations	51,966	12.3%
Revenue from vaccinations	46,621	11.0%
Revenue from microchips	8,909	2.1%
Revenue from wormers and flea control	7,424	1.8%
Revenue from surgery	56,718	13.4%
Revenue from hospitalisations	22,568	5.3%
Revenue from diagnostic imaging (X-rays, ultrasonography...)	24,944	5.9%
Revenue from blood tests	43,058	10.2%
Revenue from emergencies	30,289	7.1%
Revenue from home visits	4,454	1.1%
Total for the surgery (clinical services)	**296,951**	**70%**
Revenue from drugs	74,148	17.5%
Revenue from pet food (prescription diets and life-stage)	21,711	5.1%
Revenue from pet accessories	10,105	2.4%
Revenue from shampoos and hygiene products	8,175	1.9%
Revenue from grooming (if applicable)	13,126	3.1%
Total for shop and other services	**127,265**	**30%**
Total revenue for veterinary practice	**424,216**	

Example ➡ The veterinary practice in Figure 2 has a healthy revenue profile as it receives a considerable part of its income (13.4%) from surgery, whilst vaccinations only account for 11% of total income. To get more than 15% of revenue from vaccinations poses a significant risk, as many clients perceive this as a standard basic service that they are not willing to pay much more for. (Subsequent chapters will discuss ways of trying to change this perception held by some clients).

2. Evolution of income in comparison to previous periods

This consists in dividing the income from the current period by the income from a previous period. In this way their increase or decrease can be calculated as a percentage.

Let's imagine that we are analysing the monthly evolution of the income of a veterinary practice over the first quarter of the year.

Figure 3. Quarterly evolution of income.

Breakdown of income from a veterinary practice (fictitious data)	January 2009	February 2009	March 2009	Cumulative total January-March 2009
Revenue from consultations	3,061	3,367	4,585	11,013
Revenue from vaccinations	2,746	3,021	3,994	9,761
Revenue from microchips	525	577	800	1,902
Revenue from wormers and flea control	437	481	684	1,602
Revenue from surgery	3,341	3,675	4,258	11,274
Revenue from hospitalisations	1,329	1,462	2,224	5,016
Revenue from diagnostic imaging (X-rays, ultrasonography…)	1,469	1,616	2,561	5,647
Revenue from blood tests	2,536	2,790	3,884	9,210
Revenue from emergencies	1,784	1,963	1,600	5,347
Revenue from home visits	262	289	250	801
Total for the surgery (clinical services)	**17,490**	**19,242**	**24,840**	**61,573**
Revenue from drugs	4,367	4,805	5,328	14,500
Revenue from pet food (prescription diets and life-stage, etc)	1,279	1,407	1,206	3,892
Revenue from pet accessories	595	655	794	2,044
Revenue from shampoos and hygiene products	482	530	643	1,654
Revenue from grooming (if applicable)	773	851	532	2,156
Total for shop and other services	**7,496**	**8,247**	**8,503**	**24,245**
Total revenue for veterinary practice	**24,986**	**27,489**	**33,343**	**85,818**

We can carry out this analysis for different periods:

We could compare one month with the previous one (for example March 2009 with February 2009, figure 4).

- Or compare one month with the same month of the previous year (March 2009 with March 2008, figure 5).
- Or compare the cumulative annual total (from 1st January to the date of the analysis) with the cumulative total of the same period in the previous year, (figure 6).

Figure 4. One month with the previous one.

Breakdown of income from a veterinary practice (fictitious data)	February 2009	March 2009	% of growth
Revenue from consultations	3,367	4,585	36.2%
Revenue from vaccinations	3,021	3,994	32.2%
Revenue from microchips	577	800	38.6%
Revenue from wormers and flea control	481	684	42.2%
Revenue from surgery	3,675	4,258	15.9%
Revenue from hospitalisations	1,462	2,224	52.1%
Revenue from diagnostic imaging (X-rays, ultrasonography..)	1,616	2,561	58.4%
Revenue from blood tests	2,790	3,884	39.2%
Revenue from emergencies	1,963	1,600	-18.5%
Revenue from home visits	289	250	-13.4%
Total for the surgery (clinical services)	**19,242**	**24,840**	**29.1%**
Revenue from drugs	4,805	5,328	18.6%
Revenue from pet food (prescription diets and life-stage)	1,407	1,206	-14.3%
Revenue from pet accessories	655	794	21.3%
Revenue from shampoos and hygiene products	530	643	21.3%
Revenue from grooming (if applicable)	851	532	-37.5%
Total for shop and other services	**8,248**	**8,503**	**3.1%**
Total revenue for veterinary practice	**27,489**	**33,343**	**21.3%**

Figure 5. One month compared to the same month of the previous year.

Breakdown of income from a veterinary practice (fictitious data)	March 2008 (monetary units)	March 2009 (monetary units)	% of growth
Revenue from consultations	3.890	4.585	17.9%
Revenue from vaccinations	3,367	3,021	18.6%
Revenue from microchips	765	577	4.6%
Revenue from wormers and flea control	589	481	16.1%
Revenue from surgery	4,017	3,675	6.0%
Revenue from hospitalisations	1,821	1,462	22.1%
Revenue from diagnostic imaging (X-rays, ultrasonography…)	1,734	1,616	47.7%
Revenue from blood tests	3,554	2,790	9.3%
Revenue from emergencies	1,893	1,963	-15.5%
Revenue from home visits	345	289	-27.5%
Total for the surgery (clinical services)	**21,975**	**24,840**	**13%**
Revenue from drugs	4,985	5,328	12.3%
Revenue from pet food (prescription diets and life-stage)	1,389	1,206	-13.2%
Revenue from pet accessories	435	794	82.6%
Revenue from shampoos and hygiene products	589	643	9.1%
Revenue from grooming (if applicable)	717	532	-25.8%
Total for shop and other services	**8,115**	**8,503**	**4.8%**
Total revenue for veterinary practice	**30,090**	**33,343**	**10.8%**

Ejemplo ➡ In the first quarter of the year the total revenue for clinical services at the practice increased by 5.7% (figure 6), whereas in contrast the revenue from blood tests in particular decreased by 2.2%. This trend shows that something is happening with the blood tests that requires our attention: Have we changed any medical protocols? Are we charging correctly for this type of service? Has this decrease been the same for all vets working at the practice or is it due to one particular vet?

Figure 6. Total to date for the quarter compared to the cumulative total for the same quarter of the previous year.

Breakdown of income from a veterinary practice (fictitious data)	Cumulative total January-March 2008 (monetary units)	Cumulative total January-March 2009 (monetary units)	% of growth
Revenue from consultations	10,309	11,013	6.8%
Revenue from vaccinations	8,923	9,761	9.4%
Revenue from microchips	2,027	1,902	-6.2%
Revenue from wormers and flea control	1,561	1,602	2.7%
Revenue from surgery	10,645	11,274	5.9%
Revenue from hospitalisations	4,826	5,016	3.9%
Revenue from diagnostic imaging (X-rays, ultrasonography...)	4,595	5,647	22.9%
Revenue from blood tests	9,418	9,210	-2.2%
Revenue from emergencies	5,016	5,347	6.6%
Revenue from home visits	914	801	-12.4%
Total for the surgery (clinical services)	**58.234**	**61,573**	**5.7%**
Revenue from drugs	13,211	14,500	21.4%
Revenue from pet food (prescription diets and life-stage)	3,681	3,892	5.7%
Revenue from pet accessories	1,153	2,044	77.3%
Revenue from shampoos and hygiene products	1,561	1,654	6.0%
Revenue from grooming (if applicable)	1,900	2,156	13.5%
Total for shop and other services	**21,505**	**24,245**	**12.7%**
Total revenue for veterinary practice	**79,739**	**85,818**	**7.6%**

3. Comparison of actual income gained versus the target/budget

We have to measure whether we are meeting income targets that had been set before the start of the period. Obviously the prerequisite for doing this analysis is to have prepared a revenue forecast where the annual targets for the practice are outlined.

Analysis of practice expenditure

Once the income has been analysed, the next step is to analyse the different items of expenditure at the practice during the period being studied. Again, there are several format options for the presentation of expenditure. In the author's experience, the following format can be used by most veterinary practices.

Figure 7. Veterinary practice expenses.

Detail of the expenses of a veterinary practice (fictitious data)	(monetary units)	% against total income[1]
Purchases (usage) of consumables used in consultations, surgery, hospitalisation and the laboratory	37,161	8.8%
Purchases (usage) of shop stock: pet food, drugs, accessories etc.	52,815	12.5%
Grooming purchases (shampoos, groomer commission, etc.) (if applicable)	11,878	2.8%
Variation from inventory[2]	—	—
Total practice purchases	**101,854**	**24.1%**
Salaries of employed vets (not including partners) (total salary cost, including national insurance contributions)	70,542	16.6%
Salaries of partner vets (market salary)[3]	41,027	9.7%
Total salary costs for vets	**111,569**	**26.3%**
Nurses salaries (total cost to the business)	42,422	10.0%
Salaries of administrative personnel (total cost to the business)	22,059	5.2%
Total wage bill for non-veterinary staff	**64,481**	**15.2%**
Total wage bill	**176,050**	**41.5%**
Establishment (rent, utilities, general maintenance)	7,200	1.7%
"Opportunity cost of rental" (if the premises are owned and the owner is not receiving a rent)	30,000	7.1%
Equipment expenses (leasing, maintenance and consumables)	12,345	2.9%
Repayments or reinvestment (facilities and equipment)	25,453	6.0%
Administrative expenses (office, software licences, insurance, taxes, bank charges	16,466	3.9%
Advertising, marketing and communication	8,018	1.9%
Total operational expenses of the practice	**99,482**	**23.5%**
Financial expenses (interest from leasing)	1,876	0.4%
Financial expenses (interest from loans, mortgage)	3,224	0.8%
Total financial costs	**5,100**	**1.2%**
Total expenses of the practice	**382,486**	**90.2%**

[1]Remember that in this example the total annual revenue of the practice was 424, 216 (monetary units).
[2]We will use this adjustment only when very significant increases or decreases have occurred in the level of practice stock over the period.
[3]A market salary is what the partner would receive depending on their experience and responsibility if they worked as an employee at another practice.

Note that the different expenditure items are shown not just as an absolute value in **monetary units**, but are also expressed as a percentage against total practice revenue.

Purchases

Firstly, the purchases of consumables used at the practice, products sold (including drugs) and the materials or expenses related to other services like the groomer must be detailed.

Technically, we should not calculate the purchases but the **usage** (i.e. only consider the purchase cost of those products that have actually been sold during the period). Given the practical difficulty of making this calculation, an acceptable simplification would be to use the data for total purchases for the period. This approach will work reasonably well as long as there have been no important variations in stock levels over the period (e.g. when a large product order is placed at the end of the year in order to take advantage of a special offer). In that case we should adjust the expenses with a line called **"stock variation".**

Purchases of a typical veterinary centre vary between 20 and 25% of total income.

Wage bill

If they have anything at all in common, wage costs are the main item of expenditure in almost all veterinary practices in the world. When we talk about wage costs we are not referring just to those wages paid to employees but the total expense for the business : gross wages, national insurance contributions, benefits in kind and other related items.

Wtih regard to the owner or owners of the practice, we must also include them in the salary and wages cost centre. It would be logical to give them a market salary, i.e. similar to that which they would get in another practice (as an employee with the same knowledge, experience and hours).

In well-managed practices aspiring to reach reasonable levels of profitability (around 15% of profit against turnover) it is essential to ensure that wage costs do not exceed 40-45% of the total turnover of the practice. Higher figures indicate low productivity on the part of the vets and/or too many staff in proportion to revenue generated. On the whole, the path to achieve this productivity objective is not to lower salaries (already quite precarious in our profession) but to increase revenue from each employee.

It is also interesting to divide this cost centre between veterinary salary costs and those pertaining to the rest of the staff. **Ideally the veterinary practice should have a minimum of two non-veterinary employees (nurses, administrators, receptionists) per vet.**

The operational expenses of the practice

This section will outline all the other expenses necessary for the normal operation of the veterinary practice.

Firstly, there are **the expenses relating to facilities:** rent (if the premises are not owned), utilities (electricity, water, telephone) and maintenance. In the case of premises that are owned, even if the owner is not receiving a rent from the business, an amount should be charged in this regard. This is what economists call "an opportunity cost". This is a recognition that the premises could be rented on the market for a particular fee and that if the owner does not receive any rent from them, in reality they are subsidising, or in some way hiding a real cost of their business.

We must also account for **expenses related to practice equipment:** rent, repairs and renewals and related expenses.

At this point it would be a good idea to **clarify the difference between the concepts of expenditure, investment and depreciation**. A business incurs an **expense** when it acquires goods or services from an external source (labour, electricity, water, telephone, rates etc). On the other hand when a business acquires a fixed asset (goods worth over a certain monetary amount, which will vary depending on the tax legislation of each country, whose value remains unchanged for over a year, like for example premises, a computer or medical equipment), we talk about an investment. Although fixed assets last a long time, they do not last for ever. Accounting legislation and business prudence dictate that these assets depreciate, i.e. an amount must be calculated in each period to reflect their gradual aging. Depreciation is not really a monetary cost (it doesn´t actually have to be paid at the end of each period) but reflects the need to reinvest periodically in the renewal of the business assets. Each country´s tax authorities periodically draw up tables showing how to calculate the depreciation of different types of assets. These enable businesses to show depreciation as an expense in their accounts and thus secure the corresponding tax savings.

The **administrative costs** relate to issues such as permits, licences, office supplies, computer software, insurance and bank commissions.

Advertising and marketing costs include all the internal and external communication activities of the practice such as the website, advertisements, mailings, signage, educational material for pet owners, events and similar activities. In other business sectors there is an unwritten rule that a business should allocate on a permanent basis 2-5% of its income on these kinds of activities, something which is still rare in veterinary practices generally.

Financial expenses

When a veterinary practice gets external funding, usually from lenders, it faces **financial expense** in order to compensate those that provided the capital funding. Typically these expenses include mortgages to buy premises, loans to meet one-off cash-flow needs, medium and long term loans to finance investments in equipment, leasing installments or other financial products.

The income statement: in search of profit

The income statement, the profit and loss account, the operating statement... these are all different ways of calling one of the reports most used by any manager of a business. Drafting the income statement is little more than combining into a single document a list of the business income and expenditure in order to calculate its profit.

Following our previous example, the income statement (abbreviated) of the veterinary practice would look like the following:

Figure 8. Abbreviated income statement.

Income statement of a veterinary practice (fictitious data)	Monetary Units	% against total income
Clinical activity (medical services)	296,951	70.0%
Shop and other services	127,265	30.0%
Total income from the veterinary practice	424,216	

	Monetary Units	% against total income
Purchases	101,854	24.0%
Salary expenses	176,050	41.5%
Operational expenses (facilities, equipment, administration, depreciation)	99,482	23.5%
Financial costs	5,100	1.2%
Total expenditure of the veterinary practice	**382,486**	**90.2%**
Profits of the veterinary practice (before tax)	**41,730**	**9.8%**

The million dollar question...

What should a healthy bottom line look like?
How much should a veterinary practice earn?

One of the questions most frequent asked by veterinary practice owners is: How much should my practice earn? Although probably the answer that the vet hopes for is a specific figure, the reality is more complex. Instead of just pulling a number out of the air, it makes more sense to define some **profitability criteria** that allow us to judge whether the veterinary centre enjoys good financial health.

- **¿Does the income from the veterinary practice cover the opportunity cost of facilities (i.e. does it pay rent to the owner for any premises or facilities that its owner sets aside for the business?)**
- **Does the income from the practice enable the owner to receive a market salary (depending on the hours worked and the type of tasks undertaken)?**
- **Does the income from the practice enable the staff to receive a decent wage at the market rate and maintain an appropriate ratio between the number of vets and support staff at the practice?**
- **Does the income from the practice provide a reasonable return on assets and on the business risk taken on by the owner?**
- **Does the income from the practice facilitate timely reinvestment so that proper maintenance of equipment and facilities can take place?**

In percentage terms, a reasonably healthy income statement (taking into account the wide variation of types of practices) could look like this:

Figure 9. Healthy income statement.

Income statement for a "healthy" veterinary practice	% against total income
Clinical activity (medical services)	Between 70% and 90%
Shop and other services	Between 10% and 30%
Total income from the veterinary practice	
	% against total income
Purchases	Between 20% and 25%
Salary expenses	Between 35% and 40%
Operational expenses (facilities, equipment, administration, depreciation)	Between 20% and 25%
Financial costs	Between 0% and 5%
Total expenditure of the veterinary practice	**Between 75% and 95%**
Profits of the veterinary practice (before tax)	**Between 5% and 25%**

One final thought on business benefits

To talk about business profits is an uncomfortable issue for many vets. It is as though having profits was somehow against good medical practice, when actually the opposite is true. Good medical practice requires skilled human resources and the use of the latest technology. Without appropriate pricing (and therefore without business profits) it is not possible to motivate and retain quality staff or reinvest in training and technology. As they often say in the United States, "good medicine is good business", or "healthy pets, healthier practices". In all his years of experience, this author has never met a veterinary practice owner who started or continues in this sector for purely financial reasons. There are probably many other ways to make an attractive return on investment that are far less demanding, less risky and less tying than a small animal practice.

Key Chapter Concepts

- In order to correctly calculate the profits of a veterinary practice, **all** activity costs must be considered, including a market salary for the owner and the opportunity cost of renting the facilities that are owned.

- When we analyse the income from a veterinary practice, it is interesting to assess both the **quality** (relative importance of each line of income) as well as the **trend** over time.

- The salaries and related costs are the greatest item of expenditure on the income statement of a veterinary practice. If we can make sure that they will not exceed 40-45% of income, the economic viability of our business will be virtually assured.

- Business profit is not something bad or wicked for a veterinary practice. It is the path that must be taken in order to achieve good medicine and an investment in skills, people and equipment. Few professions have invested so much for so little return.

Putting theory into practice

How many patients should I see daily in order to at least cover my costs and not lose money? *(Break-even analysis)*

Fixed costs and variable costs

Now we will analyse a veterinary practice with a cost structure like that in Figure 7. The total annual costs amounted to 382,486 (monetary units), which were divided between a series of fixed costs and others of a variable nature.

Variable cost

This is one that increases or decreases in the short-term with variations in the level of business activity. In the case of veterinary practices, the variable cost par excellence (virtually the only one) is the purchase of consumables and products for the shop (including drugs), and the groomer (if applicable). Following the example in Figure 7, the variable costs of the practice (equivalent to purchases) would amount to 101,854 (monetary units).

Fixed cost

This is one that does **not** increase (in the short term) despite a rise in the level of sales or production in a business (some typical examples in a veterinary practice would be rents, depreciation, the wages for the majority of employees, electricity, telephones etc.). **In fact, veterinary practices are businesses with predominantly fixed cost structures:** their total costs vary very little regardless of the number of clients seen. This feature means that these businesses are very vulnerable to variations in the rate of activity: when the number of client visits drop, losses soon start. Following our example in figure 7, the fixed costs of the practice (all except purchases) amount to 280,632 (monetary units). What is striking about this figure is that we will have to pay just the same, regardless of the number of clients that visit us throughout the year. In fact if we divide these 280,632 (monetary units) between the annual number of days open (say 275 days) we will be able to calculate the fixed daily running cost (1,020 monetary units a day).

$$\text{Fixed daily running cost} = \frac{\text{Annual fixed costs}}{\text{Number of days open}}$$

That is to say that it costs the business in this example over 1,000 (monetary units) a day just to open its doors.

The contribution margin, a key concept

Let´s now introduce another important concept, the contribution margin of a product or service.

Contribution margin = selling price – variable costs

The contribution margin is defined as the amount of money that a product or service generates for the company to help cover its own fixed costs.

Let´s try to calculate the contribution margin of a service such as the "consultation". Let´s suppose that in our practice the **average revenue** generated in a 20 minute appointment with the vet is around 69.9 (monetary units) (which would include the consultation fee with the vet plus whatever treatment or product was purchased as a result of the visit).

What would be the variable costs associated with each consultation? Strictly speaking, we would just be talking about those costs generated from the mere fact of holding a consultation and that would not be incurred if the consultation did not take place. For example, the cost of the products and treatments administered to the patient. **Not** so the salary costs of the vet or the cost of the facilities as they would be incurred anyway, independently of holding, or not holding, that consultation. In the case of our example, a search in the business management programme used at the practice enables us to find out that throughout the year there were 6,075 patient consultations. Therefore, if we divide the total variable costs of the practice (equivalent to purchases) between the number of consultations, we will be able to obtain the **average variable cost per consultation.**

$$\text{Variable average cost per consultation} = \frac{\text{Variable total cost of the practice}}{\text{Number of consultations made}}$$

$$\text{Variable average cost per consultation} = \frac{101{,}854 \text{ (monetary units)}}{6{,}075 \text{ consultation}} = 16.76 \text{ (monetary units) / consultation}$$

At this point we can return to the concept of the **contribution margin.**

Contribution margin = Selling price – variable costs

and calculate that the contribution margin per consultation at this practice is:

Contribution margin per consultation= 69.9 (monetary units) - 16.76 (monetary units) = 53.14 (monetary units) / consultation

This means that, on average, each consultation that we made in this practice generates revenues of 69.9 (monetary units), of which 16.76 are intended to cover the costs directly incurred by that consultation, and the remaining 53.14 **contribute** towards covering the remaining fixed costs of the business. Depending on the level of activity at the practice (i.e. the number of consultations), we will, or will not, be able to cover the fixed costs and therefore will, or will not, be able to generate profits.

Break-even point

We know that the annual fixed costs of the veterinary practice in our example were 280,632 (monetary units). We also calculated that this meant a fixed daily running cost of 1,020 (monetary units) a day, for each one of the 275 days a year in which the practice was open.

Linking all the financial information that we have generated so far, we are now in a position to calculate **what the daily number of consultations is that will enable us to at least cover our costs.** This is called the **break-even point**, below which we will not cover costs and therefore lose money and above which we will generate profits.

$$\textbf{Break-even point}\text{ (in daily consultations)} = \frac{\textbf{Fixed practice costs}\text{ (daily)}}{\textbf{Contribution margin}\text{ (per consultation)}}$$

$$\textbf{Break-even point} = \frac{\textbf{1,020}\text{ (monetary units)}}{\textbf{54.14}\text{ (monetary units) / consultation}} = \textbf{19.2}\text{ daily consultations}$$

That is to say, this veterinary practice covers all its costs when it reaches the 20th consultation of the day, and begins to generate profits on successive consultations.

The following table and resulting graph show the evolution of fixed daily costs, daily variable costs, total daily costs and daily income for the practice in terms of the number of daily consultations. Note how the practice starts to generate profits only from the time when revenues exceed total costs (fixed costs plus variable ones), i.e. from the 20th consultation of the day.

Figure 10. Table of fixed costs, variable costs, total costs and income between 0 and 30 daily consultations.

Daily consultations	Fixed daily costs	Variable daily costs	Total daily costs	Daily income	Daily profit
0	1,020	0	1,020	0	-1,020
2	1,020	34	1,054	140	-914
4	1,020	67	1,087	280	-807
6	1,020	101	1,121	419	-701
8	1,020	134	1,154	559	-595
10	1,020	168	1,188	699	-489
12	1,020	201	1,221	839	-382
14	1,020	235	1,255	979	-276
16	1,020	268	1,288	1,118	-170
18	1,020	302	1,322	1,258	-63
20	**1,020**	**335**	**1,355**	**1,398**	**43**
22	1,020	369	1,389	1,538	149
24	1,020	402	1,422	1,678	255
26	1,020	436	1,456	1,817	362
28	1,020	469	1,489	1,957	468
30	1,020	503	1,523	2,097	574

Break-even point → 20

Daily fixed cost: **1,020 monetary units**
Average transaction fee: **69.9 monetary units**
Average variable cost per consultation: **16.76 monetary units**

Figure 11. Graph with fixed costs, variable costs, total costs and income.

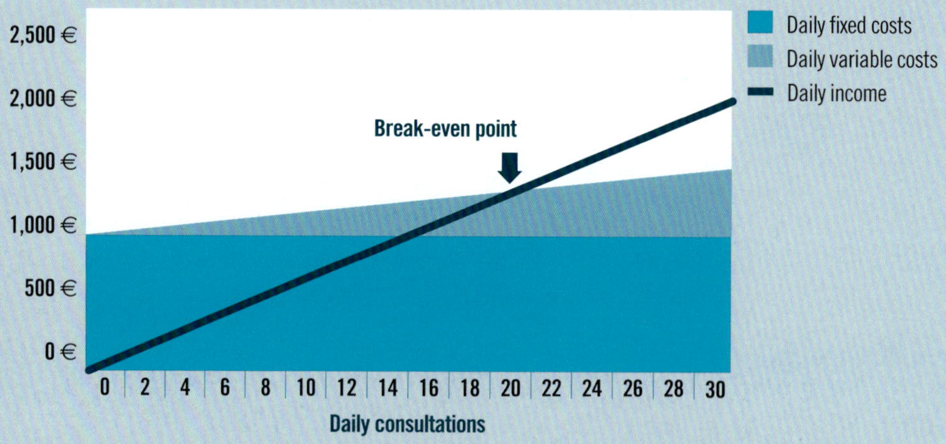

The economic valuation of a veterinary practice:
How much is my practice worth?

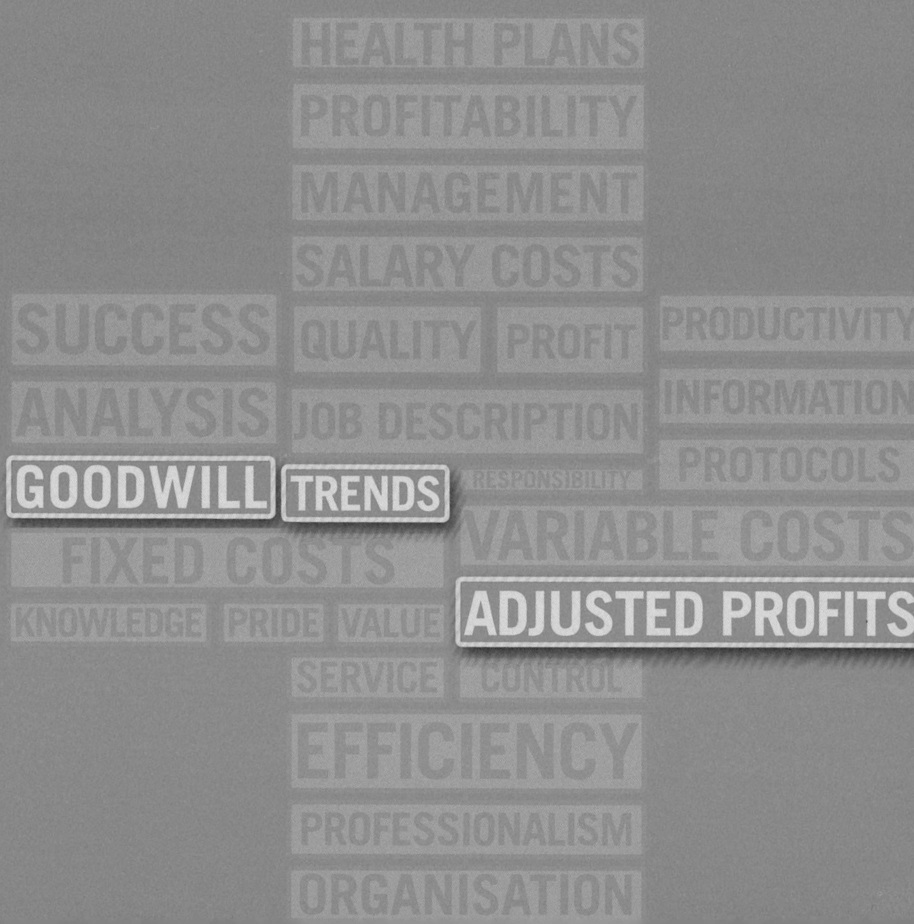

4

Why value a veterinary practice?

The most obvious situation (although not the only one) when it makes sense to calculate the value of a veterinary practice is when it comes to selling all or part of the business.

Typical examples of situations that may lead to a sale:

- When the whole veterinary practice is sold because the owner stops working (for example when the owner retires or moves away).
- When the partners in the veterinary practice decide to part company (due to disagreements or different business views). If they agree that one or more of the partners will continue with the business, an agreement has to be made for the sale of the share of the partner that is leaving.
- When the partners of the veterinary practice decide to take on one or more trusted employees as shareholders, with the aim of binding them to the business in the longer term. Then it would also prove necessary to estimate the value of the share of the business that is going to be transferred to the new partner(s).

There can be other reasons however, not necessarily related with the sale of the business, which justify the need to undertake a valuation of the veterinary practice:

- In order to make a personal financial plan for the owner or partners. In many cases, owners have a significant part of their assets concentrated in the veterinary practice, and it is important that they are aware of how the value of their business is developing.
- In order to evaluate the management of the business. Good management will result in healthy accounts and therefore in a favourable development in the value of the veterinary practice. Undertaking a rigorous financial evaluation exercise at least once every 10 years, and especially five years before the expected retirement date of the owner, can ensure management problems are detected early on with sufficient time to put into place some corrective action. There are few surprises nastier than discovering that a business, apparently healthy, has no economic value at the time of the retirement of its owner.

How NOT to value a veterinary practice: The fallacy of homemade formulas

One of the great lies that has circulated amongst the veterinary profession for many years is that there is a very simple and straightforward way to calculate the value of a veterinary practice. According to this unfounded theory, the value of the veterinary practice would be equal to the turnover of the last year[1].

There are many reasons for dismissing this theory. We will focus on some of them:

1. Empirical evidence

Recent analyses of the sales of veterinary practices made in the United States and the United Kingdom[1, 2] shows that this theory is completely inaccurate, particularly in recent years. We usually find that the valuation of goodwill (intangible assets) at the veterinary practice is set between 0.25 and 0.75 times the practice's annual turnover.

2. The value of a business is set by its profits, not its turnover

The viability of the newly-purchased veterinary practice will depend on the ability of its new owner to meet the loan payments. It is profits, and not turnover, which allows proper reinvestment in the business, ensures loan obligations are met and dividends are paid to the partners in order to compensate them for their personal and business risks.

Let's now imagine two veterinary practices with the following simplified income and expenditure structure:

	Veterinary Practice A (monetary units)	Veterinary Practice B (monetary units)
Annual turnover	750,000	750,000
Purchases	180,000	210,000
Salary expenses	285,000	330,000
Operational expenses (facilities, equipment, consumables, depreciation)	135,000	125,000
Annual profits (before tax)	**150,000**	**85,000**

Would any hypothetical buyer (in their right mind) be willing to pay the same for both businesses? Notice that both practices display the same levels of annual income.

3. Common sense: How healthy is the business?

Now let's analyse this extended comparative table featuring both veterinary practices:

	Veterinary Practice A (monetary units)	Veterinary Practice B (monetary units)
Annual turnover Year N (monetary units)	750,000	750,000
Annual turnover Year N-1 (monetary units)	650,000	775,000
Annual turnover Year N-2 (monetary units)	500,000	825,000
% of income from surgery	14%	6%
% of income from vaccinations	5%	13%
Ratio between support staff and vets	2.5	0.75
Drop-out rate of patients	8%	21.5%
Number of new patients	590	210
Parking	yes	no

With regard to all the parameters analysed, the first practice has a more advantageous position than the second. Would you pay the same for both practices just because their turnover was identical in the last year?

It is clear that the first practice, in contrast to the second one, presents a favourable income trend (growing). Income quality is also a factor to consider. The income from surgery, hospitalization and diagnostic procedures is often more sustainable over time, and less vulnerable to competitive pressure on price from other veterinary practices, than income from vaccinations. An appropriate ratio between support staff (nurses and receptionists) and veterinary staff is usually a good indicator of high productivity and quality medical care. The drop-out rate of patients tells us the practice's ability to efficiently satisfy and retain clients. The number of new patients registering reflects the growth dynamics of the business and the competitive environment of the geographic area. Qualitative issues like the design of facilities, the presence or absence of parking and the visibility of the centre in its current location will also have an influence on the valuation from the point of view of a potential buyer.

So, how do you value a veterinary practice?

An extensive range of academic literature already exists which outlines the commonly accepted methods for valuing a business in any sector[3]. There are also publications that discuss methods tailored specifically to the case of veterinary practices[1,4]. Of all these, this author prefers the use of the so-called excess earnings capitalization method, the system recommended by the North American Association of Veterinary Practice Management Consultants and Advisors (AVPMCA)[5]. This method calculates the value of the veterinary practice from its profits, making a series of adjustments that have been detailed below.

Profits: How can they be correctly calculated?

As the American saying goes, "the profits of a company are an opinion, but the cash-flow is an objective fact"[3]. This statement highlights the difficulty of calculating the profits of a veterinary practice in an objective, consistent way that allows for comparison. Therefore, we need to define a new concept that will be useful to standardise the calculation of profit, we will call this adjusted profit.

We will use the income statement of the following veterinary practice to illustrate this point:

Income statement of a veterinary practice	Monetary units	
Total income	**600,000**	
Expenditure	**Monetary units**	**% against total income**
Purchases	147,000	24.5%
Salary costs	236,000	39.3%
Operational expenses (facilities, equipment, administration, depreciations)	99,482	16.6%
Salary costs	4,800	0.8%
Profits of the veterinary practice (before tax)	112,718	18.8%

We gather more information relating to the income statement of this veterinary practice and discover the following:

- The owner, an orthopaedic surgeon with 15 years experience, had not allocated himself a salary when he prepared this income statement. His financial reward is taken from "profits". It is estimated that to employ a professional with his profile on the open market would entail an annual cost to the business of 60,000 (monetary units) (this would be the market salary for this professional).

- The veterinary practice conducts its business in premises that are owned by the father of the orthopaedic surgeon and for which a rent has never been paid until now. A quick check in a local estate agents reveals that the rent for comparable premises in the area would be 2,500 (monetary units) a month (30,000 monetary units per year).

- Depreciation amounted to 6,500 (monetary units) in the last accounting year. Remember that depreciation is an accounting concept that attempts to reflect gradual wear and tear on tangible assets over time (see chapter 3, page 55) but does not involve a real outlay of money from the business.

- When we asked the owner of the veterinary practice to provide us with the market value of the tangible assets of his business (equipment and stock), his best estimate was around 100,000 (monetary units).

- The owner of the veterinary practice has a vehicle (which is used for non-business related purposes 90% of the time) that he has financed through a lease. This lease, amounting to 900 (monetary units) a month, is paid in full by the veterinary practice (it has been allocated as administrative expense).

- The owner's wife has been carrying out administrative tasks on a part-time basis at the veterinary practice without receiving any pay. It is estimated that the cost of employing someone to do a similar job at the market rate would be around 15,000 (monetary units) a year.

- The veterinary practice has taken out a bank loan for 50,000 (monetary units) over 10 years. This loan was used by the current owner (the orthopaedic surgeon) to buy some equipment for the practice. The interest paid for this loan over the last accounting year was 4,800 (monetary units).

Now that we have this data, we can proceed to calculate the adjusted profit according to the following table:

	Monetary units
"Theoretical profit" (1)	**112,71**
+ Salary cost allocated to the owner	0
– Salary cost allocated to the owner	60,000
= Adjustment to compensate for the owner´s salary (2)	**- 60,000**
+ Cost of renting the premises allocated to the business	0
– Market rate for renting comparable premises	30,000
= Adjustment for rental (or opportunity cost) of the premises (3)	**- 30,000**
+ Cost of depreciation according to the official accounts of the business	6,500
– 5 % of the estimated value of the fixed assets of the business (approximation of the required reinvestment)	5,000
= Adjustment for accounting depreciation and real reinvestment in the business (4)	**1,500**
+ Discretionary expenses of the owner not directly attributed to the business (e.g. a private vehicle)	10,800
– Goods or services received by the veterinary practice but not paid for various reasons (e.g. 4 hours a day of administrative work undertaken by the owner's wife, not compensated financially)	15,000
= Adjustment for discretionary expenses of the owner and for unpaid services (5)	**- 4,200**
+ Financial expenses (loan interest)	4,800
– Financial income (interest from savings)	0
= Adjustment for expenses or financial income (6)	**4,800**
Adjusted profit (1) + (2) + (3) + (4) + (5) +(6)	**24,818**

The bad news for the owner of this veterinary practice is that we have gone from a "theoretical profit" of 112,718 (monetary units) per year (an attractive 18.8% of turnover) to an adjusted profit of 24,818 (monetary units) per year (a worrying 4.1% of turnover). Any well-advised buyer will make a purchase offer based on this second figure.

To reach the latter figure (more representative of the real profit of this veterinary practice), we have been adjusting the various entries:

- Setting the owner's remuneration to a level equivalent to that of the open market.
- Adjusting the cost of the facilities according to the market rental value of the premises.
- Setting the reinvestment in facilities to 5% against the real value of the fixed assets.
- Making adjustments for those business expenses or savings that are not attributable directly to the business.
- Making adjustments for the income or expenditure not related to the running of the business but to the financial decisions taken.

Tangible and intangible assets

All veterinary practices have a number of tangible assets (those that you can see and touch) like for example premises, equipment and stock. Also, some veterinary practices (if they have been properly managed) have other types of assets known as intangibles (those you cannot see or touch, but for that no less important) such as prestige, reputation, client loyalty or the ability to maintain higher price levels. Businesses in the service industry, such as veterinary practices, define most of the financial value of the business by the existence of these intangible assets.

The adjusted profit of a business is the return the veterinary owner gets against the assets of their business. One part of this return will be attributable to tangible assets, and another part to intangible assets. How can we calculate which part of the profit corresponds to which type of asset?

A commonly accepted rule is that the tangible assets of a business should be expected to return twice the risk-free interest rate. The owner of the veterinary practice has the option of investing their capital in risk-free financial assets (like for example treasury bills) with a return of 5%. Therefore, they should expect double the return (10%) when investing in tangible assets in their own practice.

Let´s return to our example:

	Monetary units
Value of the tangible assets (equipment and stock)	100,000
Loans	50,000
Net value of the tangible assets	50,000
Return expected from the tangible assets	10% (2 times the risk-free interest rate)
Return expected from the tangible assets	5,000 per annum
Adjusted benefits	24,818
Profits attributable to the return against the **tangible assets**	5,000
Profits attributable to the return against the **intangible assets**	19,818

Excess earnings, goodwill and the value of the business

Following our example, we see that part of the adjusted profit (5,000 monetary units) can be interpreted as the return demanded by the owner of the veterinary practice for the investment they have made in the tangible assets of their business. However, there is another part of the adjusted profit (19,818 monetary units), hereafter referred to as excess earnings that corresponds to another interpretation. This is the return the business owner receives for intangible assets that they have been able to accumulate thanks to the successful management of their business: prestige, reputation, loyal clients, skilled and loyal employees, etc. These intangible assets are what is usually known as the goodwill of a business. The term excess earnings tries to convey the concept of a return higher than that which could be strictly expected for the tangible assets of the business. In other words, a return drawn from the goodwill that the business has built up over the years. We could also think of excess earnings as the difference in profit between a veterinary practice that has been successfully established over several years and another practice with the same tangible assets (comparable premises, similar equipment, similar stock) that has only recently been set up.

In recently established veterinary practices, the value of the business will be very close to the value of its tangible assets (premises, machines, stock). Once the business has been longer established and builds a good reputation, establishes a loyal clientele, charges reasonable prices for its services and effectively manages its resources, its goodwill will increase in value and the valuation of the business will be clearly above the value of its tangible assets.

The excess earnings capitalization method proposes the following model to calculate the value of a veterinary practice:

Value of the veterinary practice = the net value of tangible assets + goodwill

Being:

Net value of the tangible assets = Market value of the tangible assets – business debt

At this point, we need to quantify the value of the goodwill of the veterinary practice:

How much is the goodwill of a veterinary practice worth?

Firstly, something that we need to consider is that regrettably not all veterinary practices have goodwill. Strictly speaking, only those practices able to generate excess earnings (i.e. profits above the minimum return expected on the investment in tangible assets) have goodwill.

Assuming that the veterinary practice has goodwill, its value will be calculated by applying a capitalization rate (a multiplication factor) to the excess earnings of the practice. This rate attempts to measure the risk or probability that the excess earnings currently shown will be sustainable by the practice over time. In most practices they will vary between 1 and 6, according to a series of qualitative variables that the valuer will analyse and weigh up accordingly:

Variable	Evaluation (positive, neutral, negative)	Weighting over the total of the evaluation (%)
Revenue trend over the last three years		
Adjusted earnings trend over the past three years		
Capacity of the business to retain its goodwill when the current owner leaves		
Practice location (visibility, parking)		
Quality, salary level and loyalty of staff		
Facilities (attractiveness, state of general maintenance, possibility for extension, rental terms)		
Socio-demographic profile of the area immediately surrounding the practice		
Competitive environment (quantity and quality of veterinary practices located in the area around the practice)		
Management quality (detailed and reliable financial information, well kept medical records, established protocols)		
Style of medical care (% of income from surgery, from diagnostic tests and from vaccinations)		

Revenue trend over the last three years

This will enable us to identify whether the practice has a positive trend or, by contrast, is in a state of stagnation or decline. A declining trend in income may be the symptom of a gradual loss of clients.

Adjusted earnings trend over the last three years

This is a good indicator of the quality of management at the practice. A negative evolution of profits may be due to the incorporation of new, unproductive staff, a decline in purchasing conditions or in the management of stock or an inappropriate policy of investment in equipment.

Future ability of the business to retain its goodwill

- How much income and how much of the profits of the veterinary practice are dependent on the owner who is selling?
- What future plans does the owner who is selling have?
- Is the owner prepared to sign a non-competition agreement?

Practice location

Proximity to home is still the second criterion of choice most frequently cited by pet owners[6]. Visibility, easy access and parking facilities in the vicinity are other relevant factors to be taken into account.

Quality, salary levels and loyalty of staff

A team of qualified, well paid and motivated staff is a valuable asset for any business. It is the best guarantee that the business will continue its financial performance trend after the change of owner.

Facilities

- What state are the facilities in?
- Will it be necessary to make any significant investment in the short term in order to maintain the activities of the practice?
- What are the maintenance conditions in the rental contract?

Socio-demographic profile of the area

There is a proven link between the educational level of pet owners and the frequency of visits to the vet[6].

The population dynamics of the area should also be taken into account:

- Are there new types of people?
- Are there any new estates or residential areas?
- Has the council infrastructure or its facilities changed in any way that might have a positive or negative impact on the practice?

Competitive environment of the area

- How many veterinary practices, and with which kind of profile, exist in the practice's catchment area?
- What other types of related businesses are there (specialised pet shops, dog groomers)?
- Is it likely (or viable) that new veterinary practices will open in the area?

Management quality

The quality of financial information (financial statements, information available from the management software programme) and from medical records (clinical histories) is usually an excellent indicator of the work philosophy of the practice.

Style of medical care

A high percentage of income coming from surgery and hospitalisation, or a good proportion of diagnostic tests, are indicative of a style of medical care that will differentiate the practice in the area and therefore make it less susceptible to being replicated in the future by other practices nearby.

The professional valuer will perform a detailed analysis of these variables and give them a value and relative weighting that will vary depending on their own experience. The end result will be a capitalisation rate of between 1 (in the worst case) and 6 (in the best case).

In our example, the goodwill value from the veterinary practice analysed varied from:

3 times the excess earnings = 3 x 19,818 = 59,454

and

6 times the excess earnings = 6 x 19,818 = 118,908

We suppose, for the purposes of our example, that the veterinary practice in question obtains a valuation that is medium to high by the valuer, who estimated a capitalisation rate of 4.5.

Valuation of the veterinary practice: How much is my practice worth?

At this point we are in a position to value the veterinary practice in our example:

Value = Net Value of Tangible Assets + Goodwill

Value = (Value of Tangible Assets – Debts) + (Excess earnings x Capitalization Rate)

That is to say:

Value = (100,000 – 50,000) + (19,818 x 4.5) = 139,181

Author´s comment Note that the value calculated for the veterinary practice in our example is remarkably low compared to its annual income. In fact, 139,181 (monetary units) represent 0.23 times the annual income of this practice. With this example the author certainly does not want to imply that other veterinary practices should be valued with this same rate. The point that he wanted to illustrate with this example (in addition to illustrating the methodology of the calculation of capitalisation of excess earnings) is the risk that badly managed practices have of not generating goodwill and that the value of their business may be practically the same as their tangible assets. That would be a sad result after many years of hard work and business risk.

Key Chapter Concepts

- Valuing a veterinary practice not only makes sense when planning a sale in the short term, but can also be an excellent learning exercise to check the financial health of business assets (and highly recommended at least five years before the estimated sale date of the business, in order to avoid nasty surprises with no time to react...).

- It is a fallacy that a veterinary practice is worth 1 or 1.5 times its annual turnover. In the United States or the United Kingdom it has been decades since a professional buyer would value a veterinary practice in this way. The value of a business does not depend on its turnover, but on its profits.

- The profits from a well-managed veterinary practice come mainly from its goodwill (prestige, reputation, loyalty of the clientele, involvement of its employees). A good manager is measured by their capacity to build this goodwill for their business.

- The capitalization method of excess earnings allows the value of goodwill to be quantified and, once added to the value of the tangible assets (premises, equipment, stock), will give us the total value of the business.

References:

1. McCormick, L. Contemporary issues of veterinary practice valuation and sale transactions. *Veterinary Clinics of North America, Small Animal Practice. Practice Management,* March-2006. Elsevier Saunders, pp. 297-327.
2. Sheridan, John *(www.veterinarybusinessbriefing.com).*
3. Fernández, P. Valuation methods and shareholder value creation. Academic Press, 2002 San Diego, CA.
4. Wutchiett, C. What's your hospital worth? Veterinary Economics, April 1998.
5. American Veterinary Practice Management and Consultants Association (*www.avpmca.org*).
6. AVEPA - Hill's Pet Nutrition, 2006. *Estudio de Cumplimiento (Compliance Study).*

Prices:
the 10 most common errors made by vets

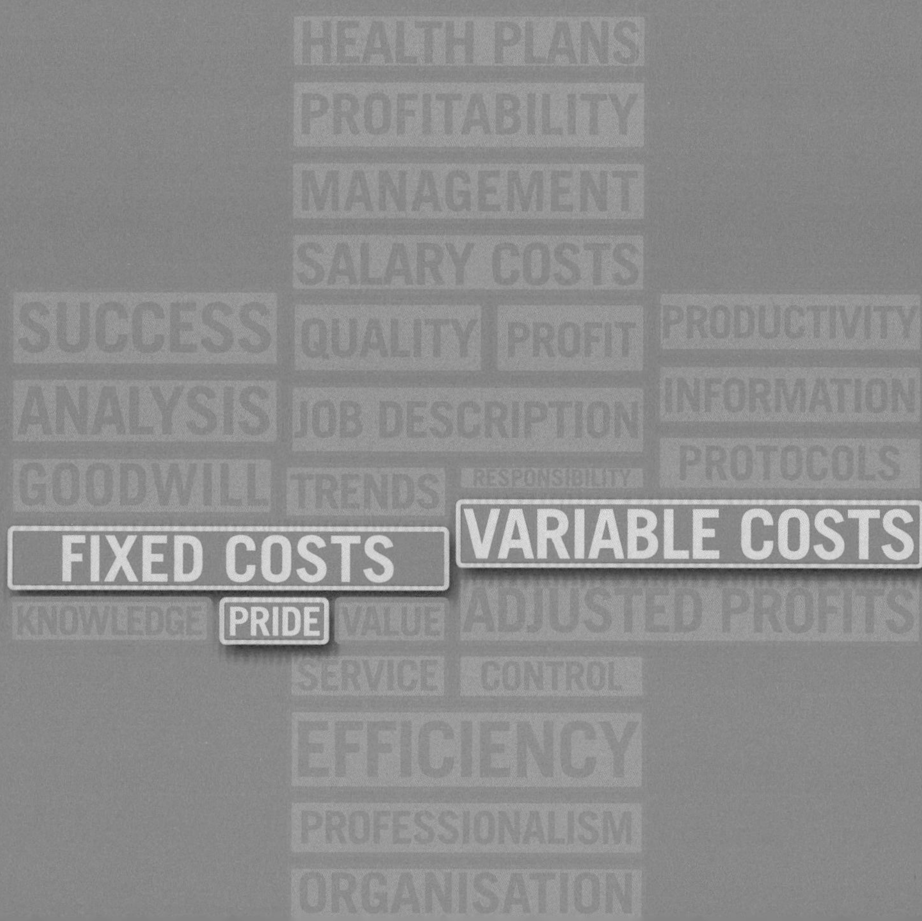

5

What is the biggest mistake a veterinary practice can make? This is a question often raised in veterinary discussion forums: congresses, management courses, informal meetings between practice owners... Probably there is no one correct answer but in the author's opinion **the greatest scourge of our sector is an incorrect pricing policy.**

Pricing is a complex problem with several possible approaches. Some argue that vets charge little because they have low social status unlike those in other professions. Others state that the excess of veterinary surgeons on the market (as we saw in Chapter 1) makes it unfeasible to charge decent professional fees. There are others who also think that the excessive demands on this profession (the vet feels obliged to know about dogs, cats, rabbits, cardiology, traumatology, infectious diseases..) generate a feeling of insecurity in the professional. This ends up resulting in low self-esteem and consequently in having a complex when it is time to charge for services. Some believe that the general ignorance of the profession about the true cost of things also does not help matters. Others even propose the hypothesis that the veterinary profession is so conspicuously vocational that money takes second place, to the extent that vets feel bad about having to charge for their services.

All these are plausible theories and deserve at least the benefit of the doubt. The reality is probably a mixture of these and other related factors. What at least seems clear is that if the profession continues to behave as it has done thus far, the best it can hope for is to obtain the same results.

The rest of the chapter offers a pragmatic view of this problem. It does not try to diagnose the causes, it simply lists a series of errors with respect to prices commonly found in many veterinary practices and suggests tools for those who want to try to obtain different results.

Error 1: To think that most clients make decisions based mainly on price

All the studies carried out on this issue show that this is not true. In a study done in the United States[1] on a thousand households with pets it was found that:

1. Only 24% of households with pets had ever changed veterinary practices over the life of their pet.
2. Of that 24% that had changed at some point, just 15% (i.e. less than 4% of total households) did it "because the previous vet was too expensive".

In Spain an extensive study[2] was also carried out which surveyed more than 1,200 households with pets. Some of the findings were:

1. Only 19.6% of the households surveyed had changed vet at some point over the life of the pet.
2. Of these, 11.6% (i.e. just over 2% of total households) had done it "because the goods sold by the practice were too expensive".
3. Price was mentioned in seventh place as a reason for choosing the veterinary practice (figure 1).

Regardless of what the studies show, one only needs a bit of common sense to appreciate that price is not the main deciding factor for most consumers. We only have to look at the restaurants, health clubs, dentists, solicitors, hairdressers, etc. In our local area to realise that there are a number of suppliers offering a range of services at varying prices. There are clients for each one of them (or the same client may choose one or the other depending on the circumstances surrounding the purchase).

Figure 1. Selection criteria for veterinary practices.

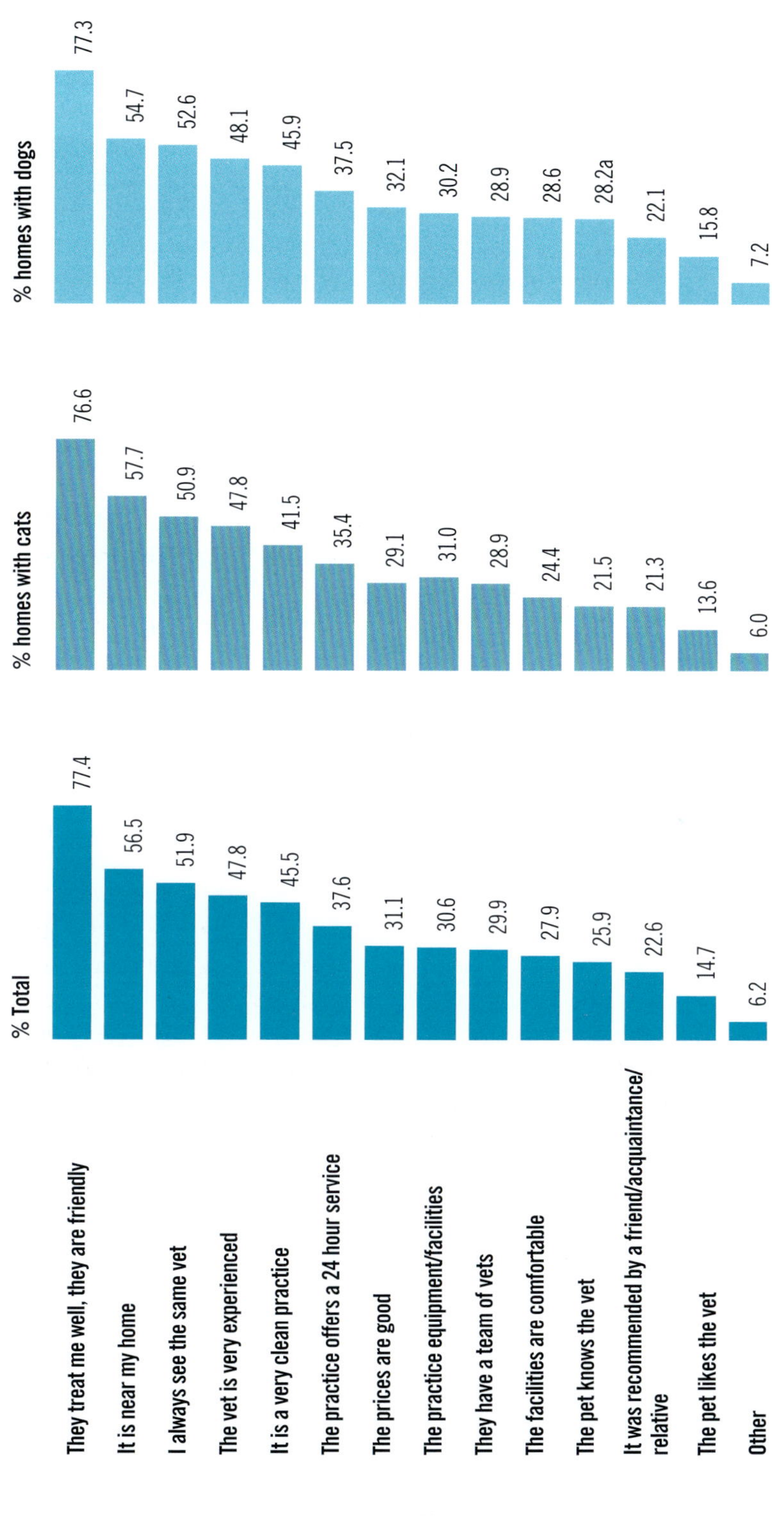

Note: The percentages add up to more than 100% because respondents were allowed to choose more than one answer.

Price is just one of the ways to compete, but fortunately it is not the only one. Moreover, the bad news for those that decide to compete on price is that in every economic sector analysed, we find the same pattern:

1. There can only be one leader in low prices (for obvious reasons: there is only room for one leader, the rest follow). Therefore, the veterinary practice that leans towards this strategy will always be at the mercy of the next one wanting to do it.

2. The position of leader in low prices is only sustainable in the medium term for those businesses that are also low cost leaders. This is a key point that many vets struggle to understand: economy of scale. In sectors with high fixed costs (like veterinary medicine), the large businesses (i.e. those that have more clients and therefore higher turnover) end up having cost advantage over the smallest ones. This happens because these larger practices or hospitals can dilute their fixed costs (website, advertising, reception, administrative costs, equipment) between a much larger number of clients.

This is not to argue that price is not important to customers.

In fact, even for those customers whose decisions are based on other factors, price is a relevant question because everyone likes to think they use their money wisely.

Error 2: Not understanding the nature of the running costs of a veterinary practice

Mark Oppermann[3] proposed a very interesting method to understand the real cost of providing a veterinary service. Most services provided in a practice contain three types of costs:

Veterinary costs

Let's do the following calculation:

- A. **Annual practice salary costs for all vets.** To calculate this we will need to consider the cost to the business, not the net salary received by the vets. For the salary costs that relate to the owner/partners, we will have to include, for the purposes of this calculation, a salary at the market rate (for example that of the best paid vet at the practice).

- B. **Annual total of chargeable "veterinary" minutes for the practice.** In order to calculate this figure we will set the number of working days per year and multiply it by the number of vets (including the owner(s)), by eight hours a day and by 60 minutes per hour. In the case of part-time veterinary staff, we will make the appropriate adjustment. Finally, we will multiply the number of resulting minutes by an efficiency factor of 70%. The logic of using this factor is as follows: not all the vet's working hours are directly dedicated to the generation of income. Telephone calls, case research and internal meetings are all examples of important tasks that can take up 30% or more of the vet's time. Therefore, we will multiply the total annual veterinary minutes for our practice by 0.7 in order to calculate how many minutes are actually available to generate income.

- C. **Cost to the business per chargeable "veterinary" minute.** This is the result of dividing A by B. It reflects how much it costs the practice each minute that one of its vets is available for a client.

Fixed or operational costs

Let's do the following calculation:

- D. **Annual operational costs of the practice.** For this we will take the income statement from the last full year and take the total costs of the business as a starting point. From this figure we will subtract the total annual costs for vets (A) and also the cost of supplies (drugs, pet food and other shop items). The resulting figure will represent the operating costs of the practice (nurses, administration, receptionists, cleaning, facilities, IT) that enable the vets to do their job.

- E. **Operational costs per chargeable minute of the vet's time.** As the reader may have already guessed, this figure is the result of dividing D by B. Its interpretation is how much it costs the practice to provide support in terms of infrastructure (facilities, support staff, etc.) for each vet for every minute that they are working for the clients.

Variable costs (cost of supplies)

This refers to the cost of drugs, swabs, vials, wormers, flea control, pet food and all the other things we use to provide a veterinary service. We must keep in mind that the cost of these supplies is not just the cost of buying them but also the financing cost to the practice (the money invested in this stock could have been invested in a bank account paying out interest), the cost of stock losses and things going out of date (it is inevitable that a certain percentage of our stocks will be lost or will expire).

Figure 2 shows the calculation of veterinary costs and operational costs for a medium-sized veterinary practice, based on a fictitious income statement (but that could reflect the reality in many practices). The reader is encouraged to adjust these calculations using real figures from their own practice and to reflect on the result... Are we charging enough for every minute of our vets´ time?

Figure 2 (a). Income statement.

Total annual income	450,000	%
1) Vet salary costs (3.5 people) (A)	112,500	25%
2) Purchase of supplies (drugs, pet food, consumables)	103,500	23%
3) Fixed operational costs (D) (facilities, utilities, non-veterinary staff)	166,500	37%
Profit	**67,500**	**15%**

Figure 2 (b): Cost per minute of the vet's time.

Number of vets (including owner)	3.5
Working days per year per vet	225
Working hours per year per vet	1,800
Working minutes per year per vet	108,000
Efficiency factor (% of strictly chargeable time)	70%
Actual chargeable minutes of veterinary time per year (total for practice)	264,600
Salary cost to the practice per actual chargeable minute of veterinary time	0.43
Operational cost per actual chargeable minute of veterinary time	0.63
Total cost to the practice of each chargeable minute of veterinary time	**1.06**

Note: this calculation only reflects the cost of the service, without any room for profits (margin) and without adding VAT.

Error 3: To make prejudgments about our clients and make financial decisions on their behalf

A very common mistake among vets is to prejudge how much an owner is willing to invest in the health of their pet based on their appearance. Judgments are made according to the way the owners are dressed, the car they drive or the area where they live. No studies have shown a correlation between the level of income and the willingness to spend more on the health of the pet. **The key is in the affective bond between the owner and their pet.** Vets should not be judges of the affective bond between clients and their pets nor their financial advisors. Clients want to make informed decisions. What they ask of us is that we inform them of the options available and, if possible, recommend one.

A revealing experiment was done in the United States[4], in which a clinical case was proposed to a group of vets. Half the participants were told that the pet owner was an elderly widow of modest means, whilst the other half were told that the owner was a young professional.

Next the vets were asked to prepare a treatment plan for the patient, and an estimate for the client. The interesting thing about this experiment is that the vets varied significantly in their **clinical** approach to the case based on the information they had available about the **pet owner**. That is to say non-clinical considerations prevailed over clinical ones. Were these vets behaving like clinical vets, or like veterinary economists?

Error 4: To mistake value with price, spending too much time talking about price and very little communicating value

Put simply, we could say that most financial decisions taken are based on two criteria:

- Value (what we get if we make that decision). This can be seen in terms of receiving goods, solving a problem, feeling happier…
- Price (what we must pay if we take that decision). This must not be strictly considered just in financial terms but also as working time, concern, inconvenience…

If the value of a decision exceeds its price it becomes attractive and we will probably take it. We will compare it with other available options and under normal conditions will choose that with a bigger difference between its value and its price.

In the veterinary practice world, the most common error is to spend a lot of time and effort in arguing with clients (and with our own employees) about the price of services and too little talking about the value we provide in return. Figure 3 outlines a service that offers value to the client.

Figure 3. Offer of a service with value to the client.

Procedure: Cat ovariohysterectomy (example)

Pre-anaesthetic clinical exam

This involves a full clinical exam carried out by the veterinary surgeon. It involves checking the patient's weight, body temperature, heart and breathing rates. In addition, the clinical status of the patient is also determined by checking the skin, coat, mucous membranes, limbs, pads, abdomen and gastrointestinal and urogenital tracts.

Pre-anaesthetic profile

The purpose of this is to check that the organs responsible for the metabolism and excretion of the anaesthetics work properly. We will check hepatic, renal and pancreatic functions. The blood and urine of the pet will be tested to rule out anaemia or infections.

Anaesthesia

This includes the premedication, induction and anaesthetic maintenance using gas anaesthesia. The patient's breathing and cardiac functions are permanently monitored using electronic equipment.

Ovariohysterectomy

This surgical procedure consists in entering the abdominal cavity by making a midline incision. Then finding and removing the left ovary (found by the left kidney) by ligating the ovarian blood vessels, dissecting them and the ovarian ligament. Then finding and removing the right ovary (found by the right kidney) after ligating its blood vessels, dissecting them and the ovarian ligament. After that the uterine cervix will have to be located and its blood vessels will have to be ligated. Once this is done the uterine body is resected and removed. The incision in the abdominal wall will be closed by suturing all the layers one by one. By the end of the surgery the ovaries, uterine horns and uterine body will have been removed.

Post-operatory

During the post operatory phase the wound will be looked after and the patient will receive analgesia and antibiotics. Ten days after surgery the sutures will be removed.

Note: The description of this service has been written by Oscar Cortadellas (DVM,PhD) (Clínica Veterinaria Germanías).

Error 5: To give money away to clients (and what is worse, without them even realising)

It is estimated that in an average American veterinary practice, the annual amount of uncharged items can amount to more than 40,000 dollars[3].

This may be due to an inappropriate discount policy, a poor administrative system used to account for services provided, or to a combination of both.

In the case of discounts, it would be a good idea if everyone at the practice asked themselves the following questions:

1. How much money did we discount in our practice over the past 12 months?

2. Who are we giving these discounts to? Animal charities? Pensioners? Those on low incomes? Other types of people?

3. Why are we giving these discounts? For charitable reasons or because we have planned to do it that way? Are we perhaps giving them because we made a mistake when preparing the estimate? Is it because we dare not defend the way we have treated a case in front of a dissatisfied customer and think this is the way to appease them? Or is it simply because one of our employees has decided that our price is too high and is giving a discount with our money?

If we do not feel comfortable answering these questions, we must rethink our practice's **discount policy**. To have a discount policy means having the answers to the following questions in writing:

1. Who is authorised to give discounts at our veterinary practice?

2. To whom and in which specific situations may discounts be given?

3. How much can be discounted?

4. How should discounts be recorded and who should be informed when a discount has been given?

Error 6: Not giving value to time (not their own, that of the employees or that of the clients)

Some vets have serious difficulties in correctly attributing a value to people's time. To start with, they do not correctly value their own time and as a result incorrectly charge for it. Moreover they sometimes have the feeling that if they do not sell something tangible to a client (drugs, pet food, an injection) they do not have the right to make a charge. Obviously if they are unable to correctly value their own time, they will find it even more difficult to value the time of their employees and clients. The most common symptoms of those vets that suffer from this serious pathology are:

- Mismanagement of the appointment diary, taking too long with the appointments therefore triggering delays that infuriate clients and put the reception team in an awkward position.

- They never find time to have a meeting with those in their team, even when they have expressly requested it. Moreover, when a meeting is finally arranged, either they arrive late or change it at the last minute.

- They never have a set time when they arrive or leave the practice and boast of working really long days. They are obviously outraged when practice staff are not willing to do the same or when a client complains about waiting for more than half an hour...

Error 7: Not understanding the dramatic impact of an inappropriate pricing policy on practice profitability

The cost of salaries and facilities at a veterinary practice vary very little, regardless of how many clients come through the door. The fixed daily running cost of a medium-sized veterinary practice in Spain (with around 300,000 euros annual turnover) is around 600 euros a day, costs that will be incurred whether one or one hundred clients come through the door…This type of business, for which fixed costs are such a considerable part of their structure, are particularly sensitive to the pricing policy. A price reduction has a big impact on their profitability, especially when it has been observed that that the demand for veterinary services by clients is relatively "inflexible" regarding price .

The demand for veterinary services is not very price sensitive

What does this mean? What is the elasticity of demand to price? This is a measure used by economists to calculate up to what point consumers of certain types of goods or services are sensitive to price variation. We talk of services being elastic to price when a price rise in these services is followed by a greater than expected decline in the demand, or when a decrease in the price of these services is followed by a greater than expected increase in demand. Conversely, we talk of services that are inelastic to price when a price rise is followed by a disproportionally small decline in demand, or when a reduction in price produces a disproportionally small rise in demand.

Studies to date show that veterinary services are relatively inelastic to demand and that within the range of prices studied, price increases of 10% used to be accompanied by reductions in client demand of only 4%.

Figure 4. Example of two services presenting different elasticity of demand to price.

Service 1 (demand inelastic to price)

Action	Price increase of 10%
Result	Decrease in sales of 4%
Action	Reduction in price of 20%
Result	Rise in sales of 8%

Service 2 (demand elastic to price)

Action	Price increase of 10%
Result	Decrease in sales of 15%
Action	Reduction in price of 20%
Result	Rise in sales of 30%

In other words, in most Spanish veterinary practices, taking into account current prices, a gradual price increase would result in a significant increase in profitability.

Making decisions: a practical exercise[6]

Let´s imagine a veterinary practice with the following characteristics:

- 5 vets (including the owner).
- 6 support staff (receptionists, nurses and administration).
- 3,000 active patients (those who have made at least one financial transaction in the last 12 months).
- Total annual turnover of 840,000 euros.

Then, presenting the following income statement (fig.5):

Figure 5. Income statement of a fictitious veterinary practice.

		In monetary units
Revenue from medical services	**70%**	**588,000**
Consultations/ check-ups	14.8%	124,320
Diagnostic services	1.0%	8,400
Image diagnostics	4.1%	34,440
Laboratory	13.0%	109,200
Vaccinations	7.9%	66,360
Surgery	11.8%	99,280
Anesthesia	4.2%	35,280
Hospitalisation	5.8%	48,560
Treatments	3.4%	28,560
Dentistry	2.0%	16,800
Complementary therapies	1.0%	8,400
Other	1.0%	8,400
Revenue from medical products	**20%**	**168,000**
Drugs prescribed during consultation	12.9%	108,360
Flea control and wormers prescribed during consultation	7.1%	59,640
Revenue from non-medical products and services	**10%**	**84,000**
OTC products (without prescription)	2.5%	21,000
Pet food	5.2%	43,680
Groomer (if applicable)	2.3%	19,320
Total revenue	**100%**	**840,000**
Purchases	**24.0%**	**201,600**
Drugs and medical supplies	9.0%	75,600
Laboratory	5.4%	45,360
Flea control and wormers	5.4%	45,360
Pet food	3.0%	25,200
OTC products	1.2%	10,080
Personnel	**42.4%**	**355,752**
Vets	22.6%	189,734
Nurses/Reception/Administration	15.5%	130,442
Office Manager	4.2%	35,575
Building (rent/interest, utilities, maintenance)	**8.0%**	**67,200**
Operational expenses	**9.0%**	**75,600**
Equipment	3.0%	25,200
Administration/services/IT/office software	2.0%	16,800
Marketing	2.0%	16,800
External (accountants, banks, solicitors)	2.0%	16,800
"Profit" (before tax, reinvestment, depreciation)	**16.6%**	**139,848**

The owner of this practice is considering four alternative strategies to improve profitability:

Option 1

➡ **Increase prices by 20%**

An accountant acquaintance of theirs has commented that if they raise prices by 20% they can expect a decrease of approximately 8% in the number of active clients. In order to simplify our exercise we will assume that the practice staff would be maintained despite the decline in activity.

Option 2

➡ **Lower prices by 20%**

The same accountant has explained to them that this decision would attract 8% more clients. To simplify our exercise we will assume that no new employees will be recruited despite the predicted increase in activity.

Option 3

➡ **Reduce by 20% the cost of purchases**

This would be achieved through a significant improvement in purchasing conditions with suppliers and improving stock management.

Option 4

➡ **Reduce salary costs by 10%**

To convince their staff to give up 10% of their salary without reducing motivation or productivity (...). Yet again, in order to simplify our example and to better illustrate the conclusions, we are going to imagine this peculiar scenario as if it was somehow possible.

The exercise consists in ordering these four options from the best to the worst in terms of their impact on the profitability of the practice. We should take this information into account as well as what we already know about the behaviour of the demand for veterinary services with respect to price variation.

Discussion

Let's analyse the four options and their impact on the profitability of this veterinary practice.

Option 1

➡ To start with, this practice has 3,000 active patients and an annual income of 840,000 euros, i.e. an average annual income of 280 euros per patient.

If we increase the price (that is to say the average annual income) by 20% (up to 336 euros per patient per year) even if it means losing 8% of the patients (down to 2,760), the annual income will have increased to 927,360 euros. This represents an increase in income of 87,360 euros (927,360 – 840,000). The only rising costs that will be incurred at the practice with this option will be purchases (if we maintain them at a level of 24% of income will we assume an extra 20,966 euros).

In summary, this option would mean additional profits for the practice of 87,360 – 20,966 = 66,394 euros, that is to say **an increase of around 48% with respect to previous profits.**

Option 2

➡ Once again let's remember that this practice's starting point is 3,000 active patients and annual income of 840,000 euros, that is to say an average annual income of 280 euros per patient.

This time we reduce the price (i.e. the average annual income) by 20% (down to 224 euros per patient per year) but in contrast we achieve an increase in the number of patients by 8% (up to 3,240). That is to say the new total annual income is now 725,760 euros (a decrease of 114,240 with respect to the previous figure of 840,000 euros). This decrease will also come with a saving in purchases, in this case 24% of reduced income (that is to say 27,417 euros).

In short, this option represents a decrease in income of 114,240 euros from which we will subtract the savings on purchases of 27,417 euros which will result in a decrease in profits of 86,823 euros, in other words **a decrease of more than 62% with respect to previous profits.**

Option 3

In this case we will achieve a reduction of 20% in the amount of practice purchases through negotiating better purchase terms and through better stock management. This represents a saving of 20% x 201,600 euros = 40,320 euros. This saving represents a rising profit for the veterinary practice, which, by these means, **would see an improvement in final results of 29% with respect to previous profits.**

Option 4

In this option, the challenge would be to reduce the total salary cost of the business by 10%. This would be achieved by convincing the employees of the need to accept this measure without it affecting their level of commitment and motivation... Assuming this is feasible, the saving obtained would be 10% x 355,752 euros = 35,572 euros, which would mean an equivalent increase in annual profits for the veterinary practice. **This would result in an increase of 25% against previous profits.**

Figure 6. Comparative analysis of the impact of the 4 decisions on profitability.

		Option 1	Option 2	Option 3	Option 4
	Starting position	Increasing prices	Decreasing prices	Savings on purchases	Cuts in salaries
Income	840,000	928,360	725,760	840,000	840,000
Expenditure	700,152	721,118	672,735	659,832	664,577
Profits	139,848	207,242	53,025	180,168	175,423
	Improvement in profits	48%	-62%	29%	25%
	Ranking	#1	#4	#2	#3

Error 8: Not knowing how to communicate to the team the importance and necessity of a proper pricing policy

It is a minority of veterinary practice owners who have held frank and open discussions with their employees about financial issues. Perhaps that is why there is deep confusion and false expectations around what a practice really earns. The employees will see money coming in (they deal with customers, charge for services, sell products) but are probably less aware of the expenses of a veterinary practice.

Let's imagine that we arrive at a veterinary practice and carry out the following experiment. We gather all the practice staff and propose the following question: "Of every 100 euros of income that this veterinary practice earns, how many euros are final profit after discounting all the expenses of the business?". In order to minimise bias in the answers, we ask all employees to record their answer individually and anonymously on a sheet of paper.

Figure 7 shows the result of one of these "experiments" conducted by the author in a veterinary practice. The vertical axis shows the percentage of profits against income that each employee estimated. On the horizontal axis are plotted the estimated values for each one of the employees of this practice.

Figure 7. Estimation of practice profits by its own employees.

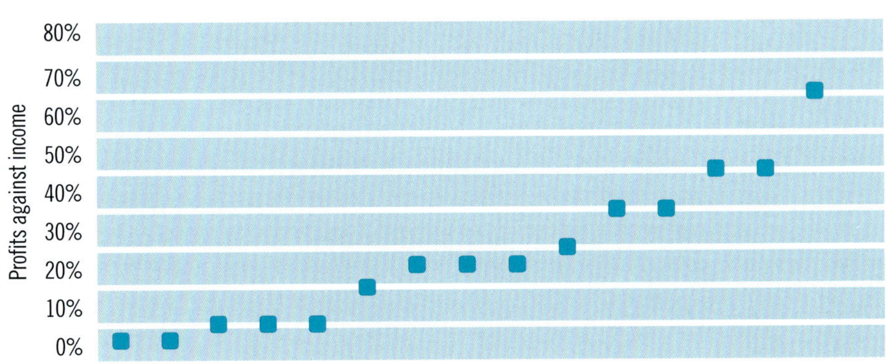

There is a remarkable disparity in employee expectations in this practice. Some believe that their practice has profits close to 5%, others of 10-15%, others of 25-30%... and there is even someone who is convinced that the practice makes a 70% profit.

Let's pause for a moment on the latter employee, the one who thinks that their practice is a highly lucrative business. What do we think the attitude of this person will be regarding the following issues?

- Level of prices at the practice.
- Discount policy at the practice.
- The importance of controlling costs (stock, consumables).
- The importance of managing payments effectively (following-up unpaid invoices, minimising non-payments made by mistake).
- Expectations of salary reviews.

We'll leave the reader to draw their own conclusions...

To avoid these kinds of situations arising, the owner(s) must lose the fear of talking about money with their team. If no-one explains to the employees what the real profitability of the business is, they will create their own expectations (as seen in figure 7). Without going to the extreme of "open book management" (i.e. sharing all the financial information of the business with employees) which is advocated by some, there are ways to focus employee expectations. Practice management courses and articles in specialised journals can be an excellent resource for this purpose.

Error 9: Victim mentality (constantly complaining of how bad the profession is without asking themselves what can I do to improve it)

Some veterinarians believe that "our real competitor is the poor service we offer in our practices". Others, however, attribute all the ills of the profession to "external forces" against which nothing can be done: the government, the universities, the RCVS, the clients, the other vets...

Everyone will act (or not) in accordance with their views on this matter. What has been objectively demonstrated (Chapter 1, page 19) is that veterinary practices still have a long way to go until they routinely use good business management practices.

Error 10: Thinking that profitability and good medical care are incompatible

Talking about business profits is something that is uncomfortable for many vets. It would seem as though financial benefits are in conflict with good medical practice, when in reality the opposite is often true. Good medical practice requires qualified personnel and the use of the latest technology. Without proper pricing (and therefore without business profits) it is not possible to motivate and retain quality staff or reinvest in training and technology. As is often said in the United States "good medicine is good business" or "healthy pets, healthier practices". Our clients, our employees, our families and ourselves deserve the same respect and dedication as our patients... We all take for granted that good medical care is an obligation inherent to the veterinary practice. What about the rest? What about our responsibilities as a service provider, as employer, and as an investor?

Key Chapter Concepts

- Vets are more obsessed about the prices they charge for their services than their own clients. Clients are more concerned about the health of their pets.
- The owner of the veterinary practice should calculate, at least once, how much every minute of the veterinary service they offer costs. This calculation will change their view about prices.
- Clients have both the right and the desire to make an informed decision about the health of their pet. The obligation of the vet is to inform and make recommendations about the best medical options available, not to manage their clients´ personal finances.
- The less the value of a service is explained, the more important the price becomes.
- Many veterinary practices lose thousands of euros every year in the form of random discounts or charging mistakes.
- The advantage of working with high prices is that it motivates and obliges the practice to offer a quality service in line with the expectations raised in the client.

References

1. AAHA, Hill's. The Path to High-Quality Care, Practical Tips for Improving Compliance, 2006.
2. AVEPA, Hill's. Mascotas Más Sanas Implican una Clínica Más Rentable (Healthier pets mean more profitable practices), 2007.
3. Opperman, M. *The Art of Veterinary Practice Management.* Veterinary Medicine Publishing Group, 1999.
4. Cron, W *et al.* Impact of Management Practices and Business Behaviors on Small Animal Veterinarians' Incomes. JAVMA, nº 217, 2000.
5. Brown J. *et al.* The current and future market for Veterinarians and veterinary medical services in the United States. JAVMA, nº 215, 1999.
6. Mercader, P. Los honorarios profesionales de los veterinarios en España: una patología crónica (Profesional veterinary salaries in Spain: a chronic pathology), Merial Journal Report. Nº2/II, 2008.

The big challenge:
to organise, motivate, appraise and remunerate the team at the veterinary practice

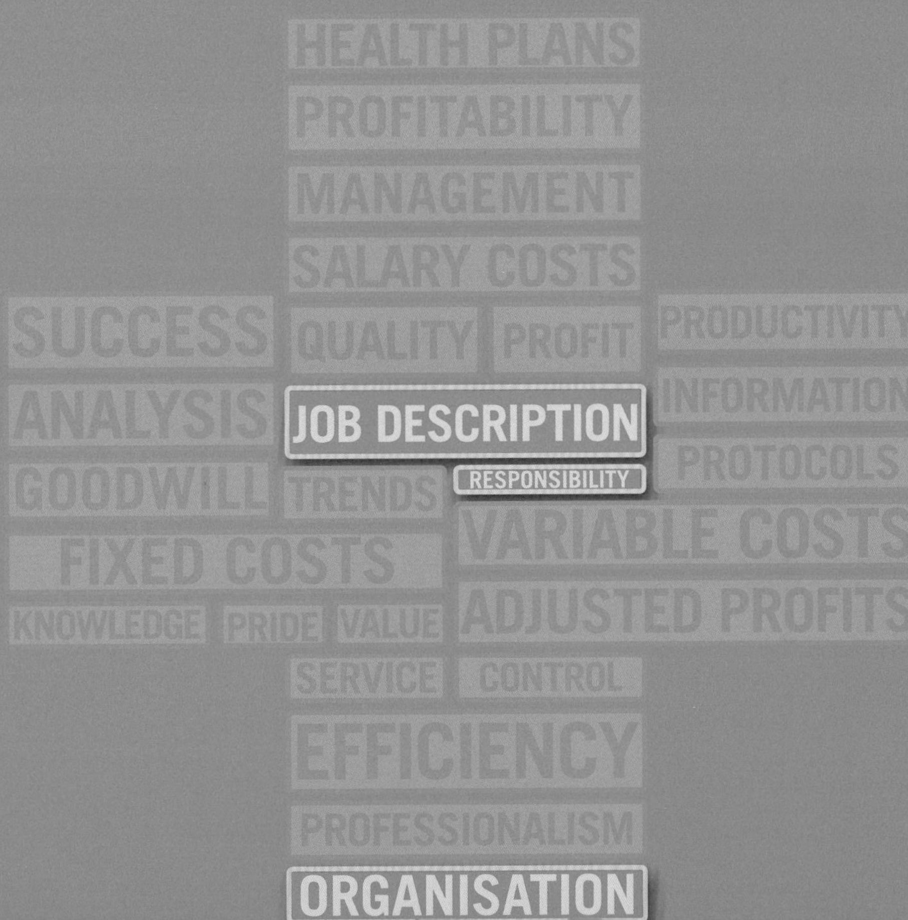

6

As a veterinary practice gets busier, it goes from being an activity carried out by a lone professional to a small business. During this transition, the real challenge for its owner is not so much to do certain things themselves as to make their team do them. What really distinguishes a good owner-Principal of a veterinary practice is their ability to organise, motivate, evaluate and appropriately remunerate their team.

In this chapter we will develop a sequential model for the management of a veterinary practice's human resources.

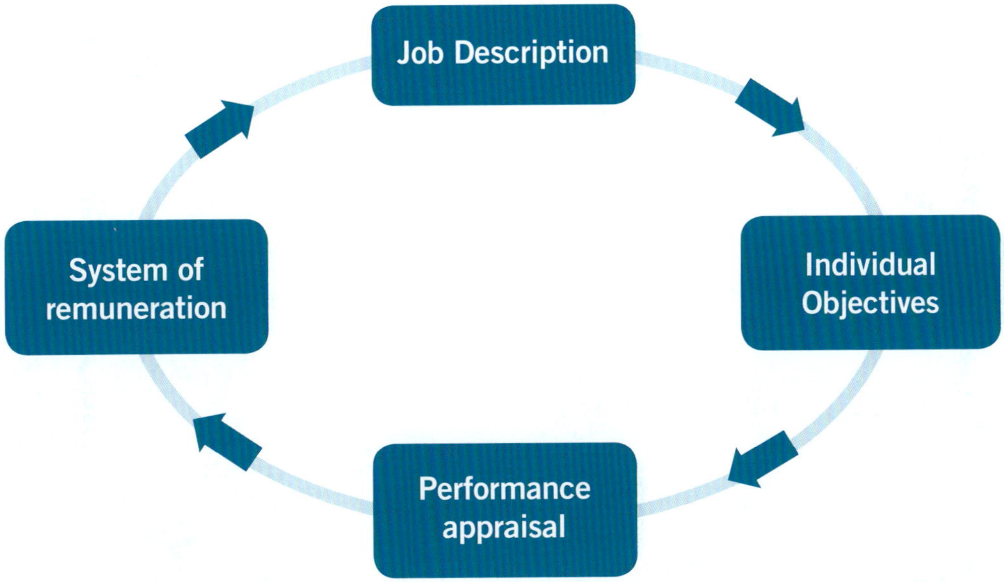

Job Descriptions

A basic tool for organizing the work of the veterinary practice team is the job description. Its main purpose is to specify the employee´s responsibilities in a formal way, looking for a balance between their expectations and the needs of the business.

Figure 1 shows a job description for the position of Receptionist in a fictitious veterinary practice.

A good job description should include the following sections:

Organisational structure

- To whom does the employee report?
- Who is their line manager in the business, i.e. who will supervise and appraise their work?

It is important to establish these points since the job description will become a kind of "contract" between the employee and their supervisor, defining the framework for evaluation (and on occasions their remuneration). Any review of a job description ought to be agreed by the supervisor and the person being supervised, and signed by both.

General purpose of the job description

This is a generic description of the ultimate aim of this post within the business. The reason for outlining this general purpose is to avoid the bureaucratic behaviour displayed by some employees who refuse to undertake particular tasks that are not specifically described in the job description. For this reason, this section of the job description emphasises the overall purpose of the job rather than describing specific tasks. For example, if the role of a receptionist is "to ensure customer satisfaction in all non-medical aspects of the visit to our practice", it is easier to understand that a good receptionist should help an elderly client to carry a large bag of pet food to their car, regardless of whether or not carrying things is written into their job description.

Job Description

Position: receptionist.

Responsible to: the manager of the veterinary practice.

General purpose and objective of post

To play an important role in the way that clients perceive the quality of services provided, whilst at reception or on the telephone.

To have responsibility for answering the telephone promptly and efficiently, arranging appointments with pet owners and maintaining a high standard of cleanliness and tidiness in the reception area. To have responsibility for managing key information to enable pet owners to know and understand the services offered by the practice.

To have an important role in the management of administrative services provided (estimates, invoicing and payments).

Main responsibilities

Administration

- Maximise the number of appointments, optimising the appointment book.
- Keep the information updated about the services provided by the practice and make it available to clients.
- Manage the system of booster and check-up reminders with clients.
- Keep client information constantly updated.

Finance

- Ensure that all services provided at the practice are invoiced and paid for.
- Minimize the number of unpaid accounts, promptly reporting them to management and following them up with clients.

Customer care

- Be attentive to pet owners who are waiting to be seen. Record and pass on messages.
- Keep the reception area neat, clean, well-ventilated and looking professional.
- Maintain a professional, kind and respectful attitude, both in person at reception and on the telephone.
- Record and pass on any complaints.
- Ensure that no clients leave the practice without either a new appointment scheduled or an updated appointment card.

Evaluation criteria

- Reception is always immaculate and organised.
- The appointment book is well managed.
- The telephone is well attended.
- Customer satisfaction (satisfaction surveys).
- Satisfaction from the rest of the team (vets and auxiliary staff).
- Percentage of boosters and clients retained.

Figure 1.

Duties and responsibilities of the job

This section offers a detailed list of the main tasks to be carried out by the person responsible for that particular job. It is recommended that tasks are grouped by area so the employee can understand and remember them more easily. The tasks detailed in the job description in figure 1 for example are grouped into administrative tasks, financial tasks and customer service related duties.

Evaluation criteria

This section is as, if not more, important than the previous one as it defines the "rules of the game" in the relationship between the business and employee. It is here where the criteria used to judge whether the employee has carried out their duties correctly are defined. Note how in the job description in figure 1 an effort has been made to make the evaluation criteria objective, i.e. transform them into measurable objectives. The importance of this is to make it clear to the team that evaluations are not based on the personal whims or opinions of management but on objective criteria. As it will not always be possible to use quantitative measures of evaluation, it is important to make an effort to explain to the team, in a way they will understand, how we have developed these criteria. Assessment criteria can have a certain degree of subjectivity but that does not mean they can be random or unfair. For example, "to present a well-groomed and professional image" is an element of the job that is difficult to quantify on a scale, but common sense tells us that the owner of the veterinary practice will evaluate their team on this point following criteria that will neither be random or unjust.

Specialised literature is available that has a full range of examples of these job descriptions, all applied to the context of a veterinary practice[1]. A practical issue to remember is that the person who best knows the details of a job description is usually the person who carries it out. It is therefore highly advisable to involve our employees in devising their own job descriptions, with our support and under our supervision. This will increase the likelihood that the job description will truly reflect the reality of our veterinary practice whilst in the process bringing about the greater involvement of our team.

Allocation of individual objectives

Once we have developed the job descriptions for our veterinary practice, they must be complemented with a list of individual objectives for each of our employees. Figure 2 offers an example of individual objectives tailored to the job description in figure 1 (receptionist).

Individual Objectives

Position: receptionist.

Period: first quarter.

Objectives

- Increase the compliance rate for booster reminders from 72% to 75%.
- Ensure that at least 70% of clients leave with their next appointment already scheduled.
- Obtain an average rating of 8 (out of 10) on the question that relates to reception in the satisfaction surveys from new clients.
- Keep the number of debts below 1% of turnover.
- Update information on mobile phone numbers and email addresses for at least 75% of the clients seen during the period.
- Correctly manage the telephone switchboard changeover.

Figure 2.

A set of well-designed objectives should demonstrate the following characteristics:

- Be specific and measurable: this will help us with their measurement and evaluation. It is not the same to say “your objective is that we have scarcely any debtors” as saying “your objective is to maintain this practice’s unpaid invoices below 1% of turnover”.

- They must relate to the employee’s duties and be within their area of responsibility: otherwise they will trigger rejection and skepticism instead of encouraging a positive response. Giving a receptionist the objective of improving the overall profitability of the business is an exercise doomed to failure. Our receptionist does not control our pricing policy nor most of our expenses, therefore it would be difficult for them to understand the direct relationship between their day-to-day job and the final net profits of the business. Instead, what this employee would find easier to understand would be the relationship between their daily job and the percentage of clients returning for boosters.

- Limited number: it is not advisable to define more than 5-6 individual objectives in any given period of time. In this way we will reduce the risk of the employee spreading themselves thinly.

- Ambitious but achievable: the objectives should result in an improvement in relation to the results obtained by the same or other employees in a similar context. However, we must set the objectives properly and avoid unrealistic goals that would be de-motivating from the start.

- Time limited: an objective only makes full sense in the context of a calendar. We must first define how often we are going to appraise our team and then give them individual objectives within the same time frame.

Performance Appraisal

The performance appraisal is a formal and systematic process in which all practice employees meet periodically with their supervisor and are assessed on the tasks they have been undertaking. The example in figure 3 shows a template usually used in formal performance appraisals.

The main features of this template are:

- List of individual time-bound objectives.

- Relative importance of the different objectives shown as a percentage.

- Evaluation of the results obtained for each of the objectives. Notice that the rating scale is not the conventional 0 to 10, but 0 to 12. The reason for this is to encourage the employees to give their all to each task, and not to reduce their efforts once they achieve an objective.

Figure 3.

Performance Appraisal Plan

Position: Receptionist/customer care | **Period under evaluation: (Q1: First quarter)**

Objective (Description)	Reference measure (Objective specification)	Result obtained by the employee	Grade (Scale 0-12)	Relative relevance (% over 100)	Score
1. Increase the percentage of boosters.	Ensure booster rates go from the current 70% to 75%.	Decreased to 66%.	0	25%	0
2. Increase the client retention rate.	Ensure that at least 70% of clients leave with a scheduled appointment (this data was not available before).	Reached 55%.	6	20%	1.2
3. Client satisfaction with reception.	Obtain an average rating of 8 (out of 10) on the question that relates to reception in the satisfaction surveys from new clients.	Rating of 8.5 given to reception in surveys completed.	12	20%	2.4
4. Minimise debts, chase debtors.	Keep the number of debts below 1% of turnover.	It remained around 1%.	10	15%	1.5
5. Improve the quality of the data in the client records.	Obtain mobile phone numbers and email addresses for at least 75% of the pet owners that will visit us during the period.	This data was obtained from 60% of pet owners visiting us.	7	10%	0.7
6. Correctly manage the changeover from one switchboard provider to another.	New switchboard to come into operation on 15th March, without disruption to service. Support staff trained in its operation.	The new switchboard started without serious problems on 10th March. The staff received training.	9	10%	0.9
				Final Score	6.7

Summary of results and observations

Final score of the performance appraisal plan by objectives

In general, a satisfactory result. The most obvious area for improvement is the management of booster reminders.

The employee overlooked the follow-up calls for the overdue booster reminders sent by post although there were some time constraints due to her having to temporarily replace another member of the support staff who was off sick.

In this way we avoid the so-called "ratchet effect", whereby some employees deliberately reduce their efforts when they reach an objective before time in order to avoid their supervisor setting even higher objectives in the future.

- Comments that provide additional information, helping to clarify both the results and the appraisal.

Practical recommendations for the implementation of a performance appraisal system

- Communicate, communicate and communicate. Reach a mutual agreement with each employee on their individual objectives and do it at the start of the assessment period. Explain the evaluation criteria (weighting, performance measures used) and the frequency with which they will take place. Explain how the performance measures will be calculated and why those, and not others, have been chosen.

- Appraisal meetings should be well-prepared. A week or two before holding the meeting we should ask the employee that is going to be appraised to prepare a draft "self-assessment". The employee will need access to the results of their performance measures to do this. This system has the advantage of further involving the person who is supervised, and making them more conscious of their results and the factors that have influenced them.

- The appraisal should be focused on the behaviour and the results, not on the person. It may seem like a subtle nuance but it is not the same to say to a person "you are unprofessional" as saying "your conduct this last quarter has not been very professional". These distinctions (and the corresponding explanations) can mark a fine line between constructive criticism and a personal insult.

- Present the individual acting as supervisor as a resource for the employee and not as a controlling figure. The skill of the supervisor lies in reaching an accurate assessment, mutually agreed with the employee, about why the objectives have not been achieved and how this will be corrected. The reasons why the desired outcome has not been achieved should be discussed with the employee. We must also consider whether the supervisor can provide any reasonable resources that the employee needs to improve the achievement of their objectives (CPD, training, better supervision, an organisational change).

In reality, the formal systems of performance appraisal are intended to ensure that each employee and their supervisor spend some quality time together. This time is used to periodically review the most important issues in relation to their job description.

At an organisational level, it is considered unlikely that a manager can properly supervise more than seven or eight employees. Therefore, if in our veterinary practice there are already more than eight people working, we should seriously consider adapting our organisational structure and defining a first line of "middle managers".

Figure 4 shows an example of a functional organisational structure, where staff are grouped by areas of work (vets, nurses, administration) led by a smaller group of middle managers.

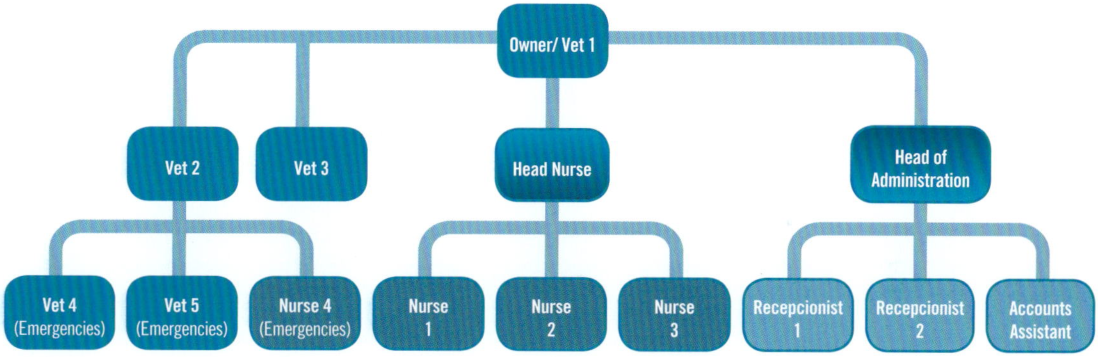

Figure 4.

Thus, the owner of this practice -where 14 people work- is supported by a small management team consisting of 4 people.

Remuneration schemes for veterinary staff: How much, how and why should they be paid?

If we look again at an income statement that is typical of many veterinary practices, we can see a series of financial ratios that help us to understand and define how much money we can use to pay our team.

Figure 5. Income, expenditure and profits of a veterinary practice.

	Income as a percentage
Income	**100%**
Medical services	70%
Shop	30%
Staff expenses	**40-45%**
Vets	25%
Support staff	15-20%
Purchases	25%
Operational expenses (Facilities, administration, IT systems, etc.)	20%
Profits	**10-15%**

On the one hand we see that the total salary cost of staff should not exceed 40-45% of business turnover. On the other hand we know that the typical staff structure of veterinary practices in many countries divides this 40-45% of salary costs into 25% for vets (including owners/partners) and 15%-20% for the remaining staff at the practice.

These ratios imply that on average each vet at the practice should generate income equivalent to four times their total salary cost (gross salary plus national insurance plus taxes). Or, conversely, that a veterinary assistant could receive a salary that cost the equivalent for their practice of, let's say, a quarter of the income generated by that person. The following table shows this ratio for various net monthly salaries for a veterinary assistant:

Figure 6. Cost of the vet's time.

Vet's fixed net monthly salary	1,200	1,500	1,800
1. Annual salary cost to the business (x 12 x 1.22 x 1.35)	23,717	29,646	35,575
2. Variable incentives (20% of fixed salary)	2,880	3,600	4,320
3. CPD expenses (courses. journals)	300	300	300
4. Discounts for own pets	150	150	150
5. Total annual cost to the business	27,047	33,696	40,345
6. Cost per hour (40 hours a week, 46 weeks a year)	14.7	18.3	21.9
7. Cost per minute	0.24	0.31	0.37
8. Efficiency (60%)	60%	60%	60%
9. Effective cost per minute	0.37	0.46	0.55
10. Charge made to the client per minute (x4)	1.48	1.85	2.21
Charge made to the client for 20 minutes (before VAT)	**29.7**	**37.0**	**44.3**
Charge made to the client per hour (before VAT)	89	111	133

Let's consider a vet whose net monthly salary is between 1,200 and 1,800 monetary units (you can follow the explanations given in the column that best represent the reality of your practice). In order to calculate the salary cost of this employee to their practice, we will first convert this net monthly salary into an annual gross salary and add the national insurance costs (1). Then we will add other costs to the practice such as variable bonuses or non-salary based remunerations like CPD or discounts for their own pets (2), (3), (4). At this point we can calculate the total cost of this employee to the business (5), which we can break down into cost per hour (6), or per minute (7). The working day of a vet does not consist solely in chargeable time with clients. Telephone calls, administrative tasks, internal meetings and time studying cases, etc. are all relevant and necessary tasks but compete with the vet's chargeable time. Let's assume that only 60% of the vet's working day is likely to be spent in consultations with clients and therefore in generating revenue (8). If we apply this factor to the salary cost per minute, we will obtain a figure for the effective chargeable cost per minute of this vet (9). Finally, if we apply the previously mentioned ratio of 4 to 1 from the table above, we will have calculated the revenue (before VAT) that has to be generated to allow those 20 minutes of consulting time to be financially sustainable by the practice. In the case of a vet with a net monthly salary of 1,500 monetary units, the conclusion drawn is that if the resulting consultation charge (consult fee) plus tests, treatments or products resulting from it do not reach 37 monetary units, the veterinary practice is not achieving the minimum levels of profitability required.

How should we pay our employee vets: a fixed salary, a variable one or or a combination of both?

Fixed remuneration schemes for vets (a fixed salary regardless of the results achieved) have traditionally been the most commonly used in non-English speaking countries. In the United States, however, variable salaries are the most commonly used[2]. In these schemes, the financial compensation for the employee is linked with the achievement of certain objectives, or directly as a percentage of revenue generated. In many North American clinics, the vets receive between 19 and 23% of revenue generated through medical services. There are many variations on this system, diploma holders tend to receive very different percentages depending on the characteristics of their specialty and the overheads their activities generate. For example, the overheads for an orthopaedic surgeon cannot be compared with those of a dermatologist, and therefore their variable salary percentage against income generated cannot be the same…

Mixed or hybrid remuneration schemes combine a fixed base salary with a bonus or variable allowance that is based on various criteria (percentage of turnover, achievement of qualitative objectives, etc.).

Advantages and disadvantages of variable pay schemes

The popularity of variable pay schemes comes mainly from the fact that they are designed to have a positive effect on the motivation and effort of employees. Another attractive feature of these schemes is that in a way they put part of the business risk onto the employee, converting them into a kind of partner. That is to say, if the business is going well and has a high turnover, the employee perceives the benefit as he earns more than usual. However, if the business is not doing well and has a low turnover, the employee will be partially affected and will receive a lower salary. This allows the business to have a more variable salary cost structure, and is therefore less susceptible to market fluctuations.

However, these remuneration schemes are not without their problems. Readers with experience in this field will probably remember unpleasant situations with employees who reacted in a negative way when they found their salaries had been linked to their personal turnover:

- Focus on quantity rather than on quality. Shorter consultations and more concise explanations given to clients.
- Overinflated bills. Tendency to run too many diagnostic tests and systematically choosing the more expensive medical options, relegating medical considerations to second place.
- Deteriorated working environment. Arguments amongst team members over who did what or whose case it is.
- Neglect of qualitative aspects of the work. In a variable turnover-linked remuneration scheme, vets perceive any non-income generating activities as a waste of time: answering telephones, training younger inexperienced staff, attending practice meetings, writing thorough clinical histories, etc.

In order to minimise any adverse effects, it is recommended that those vets who have already opted for variable remuneration schemes use balanced evaluation criteria. In other words, those that combine the quantitative and qualitative aspects of the job.

The following example shows one of these balanced remuneration models where financial productivity is integrated with other important aspects of the vet´s job:

Figure 7. Balanced system of variable remuneration.

Fixed salary	100
Variable salary	from 0 to 25 extra, depending on performance appraisal
Performance appraisal	Weighting
Personal turnover	30%
Excellence in customer service	30%
Team leadership and capacity to teach	20%
Ability to follow protocols	20%

Notice how in this example the variable remuneration has limited weighting (the highest it can reach is 25% of the fixed salary). Also notice how the criteria used to decide this variable salary component combines income generation with other "softer" criteria (client satisfaction, leadership and training of other members of the team, following internal protocols).

Key Chapter Concepts

- You have to "start the house with the foundations". In other words you have to start off by developing good job descriptions and individual objectives for all the staff at the veterinary practice.
- It is important to get into the habit of carrying out periodic performance appraisals at the practice which initially should not be linked to any variable remuneration scheme. Gain experience using this system, and generate confidence in the team regarding the evaluation criteria.
- If ultimately it is decided to incorporate a variable component as part of staff remuneration, this must be done through a balanced set of criteria that go beyond pure percentage of turnover. The criteria should be put in writing and incorporated into the formal appraisal system.
- Variable remuneration schemes are very powerful tools that affect people´s behaviour at work. It is much better not to have a variable remuneration scheme than have one that has been badly designed…

References

1. WILSON, J. *Job Descriptions and Training Schedules for the Veterinary Team.* Priority Press Limited, 2005.
2. WILSON, J. *Contracts, Benefits, and Practice Management for the Veterinary Profession.* Priority Press Limited, 2000.

Customer care
in the veterinary practice

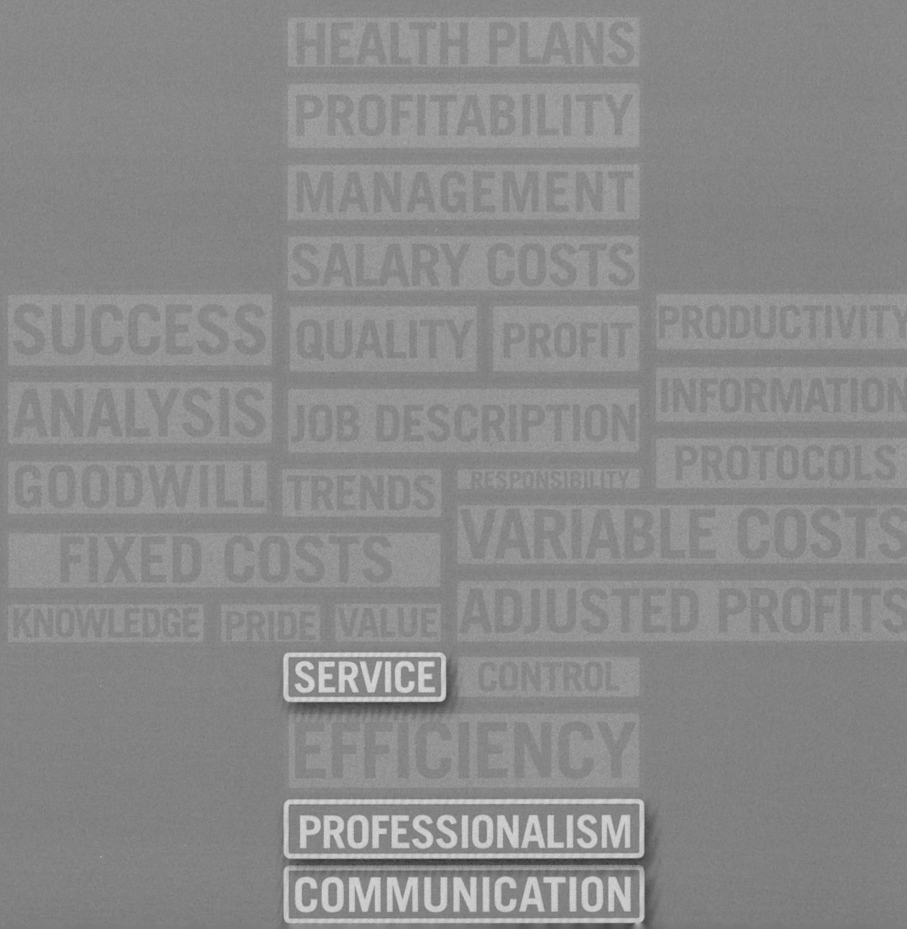

7

Most times when we go to a human hospital, we don't do it for a good reason. Apart from the birth of a baby, most of our personal experiences of hospitals are linked to complicated situations that generate a certain degree of anxiety or fear in us. Similarly, many of the visits that patients and clients make to our veterinary practice are stressful for them.

Knowing this we should set ourselves the following objectives for each and every one of our clients' visits:

1. Create a pleasant experience for them

Everything surrounding the medical care (telephone, reception, dealings with staff, administrative matters) should be as pleasant and efficient as possible for our clients and patients.

2. Give them peace of mind

We should always reassure our client that they have made a good decision in entrusting the health of their pet to us, as we will treat it professionally and with the utmost care. We want the client to perceive themselves as a responsible pet owner that does the best possible for their pet. This is usually described as "peace of mind".

3. Clearly explain the value of the service provided

The client must perceive, and understand, the benefits that they and their pet are receiving for their money, as this will have a positive impact on their level of satisfaction with our service.

Of course all of this must be accompanied by a positive outcome following the professional treatment of the medical condition that triggered the patient's visit.

Throughout this chapter we will develop a methodology which aims to achieve these objectives.

Managing the appointment book

Many experienced veterinary practice owners admit quite unashamedly that the most indispensable person on their team is a good receptionist. As well as being the face and voice of the business for clients, reception staff are responsible for efficiently managing the practice's appointment book, which at the same time has an impact on the way the work in the practice is organised.

"By appointment" or "open surgery"?

The trend towards the scheduled appointment system as the way of organising work in veterinary practices is relentless. In recent years, this system has become standard practice for the majority of practices. The popularity of this way of working is due to the advantages it offers both to the client and the veterinary practice:

Advantages for the client

1. Shorter waiting times

In today's society it is almost inconceivable that you would ask a client to wait 40 to 50 minutes to receive a service. A well-managed appointment system will help us to drastically reduce waiting times at our practice.

2. Better client and patient care

One of the biggest advantages of scheduling appointments is that we know in advance which clients are going to visit us and why. As a result we can prepare in detail any necessary information to ensure we provide the best personal attention and medical care to our clients and patients.

Advantages for the veterinary practice

1. Better organisation of work

This will allow us to spread the workload throughout the week, avoiding the typical peaks and frustrating troughs in activity levels. This will also enable us to have appropriate staffing levels at the practice.

2. Adapting the service to different client profiles or different medical conditions

Does it not make good business sense to reserve the best slots in the week for our best clients? Or to allocate different consultation periods to different medical conditions? (see example in figure 1).

Figure 1. An example of how to divide the appointment book.

Type of appointment	Diary time
Normal appointment	20 minutes
Follow-up appointment	10 minutes
Appointment with specialist	45 minutes
New puppy appointment	30 minutes
Juvenile appointment	30 minutes
Diagnostic test A	30 minutes
Diagnostic test B	45 minutes

3. Raising the professional image of the vet

Has it ever occurred to us to go and see an architect, a solicitor or lawyer without first asking for an appointment? Of course it would never occur to us because we think of these qualified professionals as very busy people, whose time is valuable and in all probability are not sitting around idly in their offices waiting for a client to suddenly decide to visit them. Following the same logical reasoning, why then do we teach our clients to do exactly the opposite? Do we want to be seen as health service professionals or as retailers where people stop by to make unplanned purchases? We should ask ourselves this question and act accordingly.

4. Proactive management of customer relations

This is another issue that is key to the efficient running of the clinical and business sides of the veterinary practice. If we decide to tell a client: "come back in a few days" or "come back next year" or "come back if Luna isn´t feeling well", when do we honestly expect that this client will return to our practice? Why leave in the hands of the client the responsibility to decide when to go to the vet?

Would not it be more logical if we, in our capacity as the **health service managers** for their pet, set the pace of the appointments? Another of the major advantages of the scheduled appointment system is that it enables us to make specific recommendations about when to return to the practice: "Mrs Smith, the vet tells me that we need to check up on Luna´s progress next week. When would it be most convenient for you to come, Tuesday at 5.30 pm or Wednesday at 9.30 in the morning?".

Two practical ideas for managing the appointment book

1 Start the appointment book with an "atypical" time. When does the reader think the client is more likely to be punctual, when we have given a time of 9 am or when we have asked them to come at 9.35 am? Various studies show that client punctuality is increased when we give them a time that is more difficult to remember as they pay more attention to it. Try to be a bit creative with the management of the appointment book...

2 Book a 45-60 minute buffer time for each vet in the middle of the morning and during evening surgery to allow them to catch up if they are running late or to use it for administrative or managerial tasks.

Do your homework: prepare for the consultation... before the consultation

The best preparation for a consultation is that which starts **before** the client and the patient turn up at the veterinary practice. To this end, it is recommended that the following routines are observed:

- Make reminder calls (or send emails or text messages to mobile phones) for all those appointments arranged more than two weeks in advance. This will significantly reduce the number of missed appointments or late arrivals by clients.
- Review in advance any areas of preventative medicine where there is room for improvement. The template in figure 2 is an interesting example of proactive preparation for the consultation.

Patient:: Date:

PATIENT HEALTH AND CLIENT CARE MONITORING RECORD

Any change of address?	No	Yes
Do we have a current email address?	Yes	No
Do we have a mobile telephone number?	Yes	No

OBSERVATIONS

			Customer Care	Vet
Does the pet have a microchip?	Yes	No		
Has it been neutered?	Yes	No		
Are vaccinations up to date?	Yes	No		
Vaccination reminders recorded?	Yes	No		
Wormers up to date?	Yes	No		
Wormer reminders recorded?	Yes	No		
Flea control up to date?	Yes	No		
Flea control reminders recorded?	Yes	No		
Protection against Leishmania	Yes	No		
Do we have a current photograph?	Yes	No		
Older pet	No	Yes		
(Older pet health plan recommended?)				

Any problems with joint movement, limping?	No	Yes
Any digestive problems, diarrhoea, sickness?	No	Yes
Any change in behaviour noticed?	No	Yes
Any change in urinary or defecating habits?	No	Yes
Any sign of coughing, sneezing, panting?	No	Yes

Dental condition	1	2	3	4	5
Body condition scoring	1	2	3	4	5
Weight					
Temperature					

Nutrition. Note type of diet		
Daily quantity		
Prescription diet recommended?	No	Yes
(Indicate type recommended)		

DATE OF NEXT APPOINTMENT

Figure 2.

A possible system for preparing for the visits could be as follows:

- Every afternoon, a receptionist or nurse could check the medical records of those patients with an appointment scheduled for the following day. Those patients scheduled for surgery or diagnostic tests would be excluded.

- Following the format proposed in the template in figure 2, any outstanding administrative information that is needed can be identified (for example email addresses or mobile phone numbers).

- Similarly, this procedure will highlight any preventative medical procedure (vaccinations, worming, neutering, etc.) in which the patient is not up to date, or where we do not have up to date information.

- The next day, these issues will be discussed with the client (in the reception area) and appropriate entries will be made on the patient's record in order to save the vet and nurses time in the consulting room.

The advantage of using of this system lies in the fact that it frees up veterinary time, allowing them to focus on the patient examination, the diagnosis and any treatment recommendations. In addition it gives the client the impression that the health of their pet is being comprehensively monitored.

Veterinary protocol for client care during the consultation

According to some, the consultation is the temple of veterinary medicine. The client's perception of our service will largely depend on what happens during the consultation and on the manner in which it is conducted. That is why it is very important to develop a client and patient care protocol for the consultation. This will help our clients to have a consistent experience in our consultations, regardless of the day of the week they come or the vet on our team who sees them.

It is disturbing to see the lack of consistency in both the physical examination of patients and the treatment given to clients in many veterinary practices. It is therefore highly significant that one of the most prestigious medical textbooks[1] devotes its first chapter to the proposition of a detailed protocol to follow during the consultation, including very specific recommendations about how to address the client. What is also significant is the large number of vets who quietly skip over this chapter in order to focus directly on those chapters that they perceive to be properly clinical.

In our case we propose the following customer care protocol during consultations:

1 Present a professional appearance
Remember that our client is unable to judge the quality of our medical procedures and therefore seeks external signs to reassure themselves. A clean uniform with the appropriate identification and an immaculate, discrete and smart appearance all project a professional image in a medical environment.

2 Greet the client in a professional but friendly manner
Introduce yourself, giving your name and position at the practice. Smile and shake hands with the client.

3 Interact with the pet from the start
Greet the pet by name, establish physical contact with it and make a friendly comment to relax the owner.

4 Apologize if we are running late

Praise clients that arrive on time. As well as a gesture of courtesy, these practices send a clear message both to the client and the rest of the team regarding the value of their time and ours. In the same vein, it is also advisable to call those clients who have not turned up for their appointment 20 minutes after the time agreed. The call must be polite and friendly, but it will help us to remind the client that a vet at our practice has spent several minutes waiting for them.

5 Use the name of the owner and the pet at least once during the consultation

This will improve interaction and demonstrate a service orientation. Even the most skeptical clients who think we pulled their name from the clinical record a few minutes before they arrived will positively appreciate our efforts as a sign of professionalism.

6 Perform a thorough physical examination, always explaining to the owner what we are doing and what our findings are

We often forget that what seems obvious to us is a mystery to our clients, especially if we do not exteriorise it. Half a minute spent in silence inspecting the inner ear of the pet can be an eternal wait for an apprehensive client.

7 Always provide some written information

This improves customer understanding, makes sure clients remember our veterinary practice and, in short, increases the perception of value regarding the service received. The following consultation report (figure 3) is an excellent educational tool for clients.

Furthermore, the report's use has a valuable secondary purpose: to provide standard and systematic guidelines for all the vets at the practice when carrying out physical examinations of patients.

8 Make eye contact with the client, especially when we are delivering an important message

It is important to avoid writing or staring at the computer when we are making a health recommendation to a client.

Seixal Veterinary Hospital

Consultation report Date ___/___/___

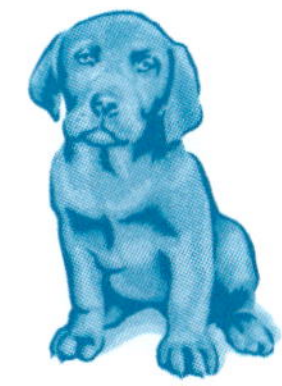

Name ________________ Date of birth ____________ Sex ____

Owner´s name ________________ Telephone Number ____________

Microchip Yes ☐ Still doesn´t have one ☐

Preventative care:

		Up to date	Done today	Not done
Vaccinations:	Annual vaccination	☐	☐	☐
	Rabies vaccine	☐	☐	☐
Wormers		☐	☐	☐
Flea / tick control		☐	☐	☐
Heartworm prevention		☐	☐	☐

Clinical examination:

Skin and coat
☐ Normal
☐ Alterations

Limbs
☐ Normal
☐ Alterations

Heart and lungs
☐ Normal
☐ Alterations

Gastro-intestinal system
☐ Normal
☐ Alterations

Eyes
☐ Normal
☐ Alterations

Ears
☐ Normal
☐ Alterations

Uro-genital and mammary glands
☐ Normal
☐ Alterations

Mouth and teeth
☐ Normal
☐ Alterations

Body condition:

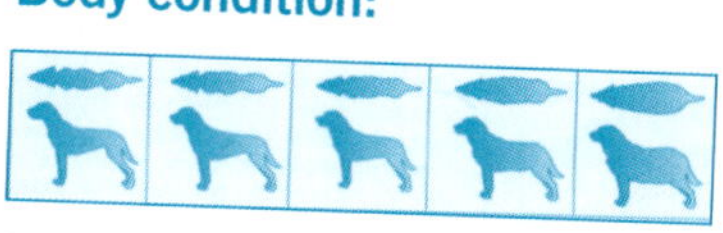

Diagnosis and recommendations

____

____

____

____

____

Figure 3. Consultation report (copyright of HV do Seixal, www.hospitalveterinariododeixal.com).

9 Combine verbal explanations with visual media whenever possible

It has been demonstrated that the use of drawings, illustrated atlases, articulated models, videos, etc. significantly improves levels of client understanding (and therefore the likelihood that they will accept and remember what is being said). Nowadays there are a number of high quality communication tools accessible to those vets who want to use them.

10 Use layman's terms but without lapsing into trivialities or inaccuracies

A common mistake among younger vets is to try to impress clients with sophisticated terminology in the false belief that this will reflect positively on their professional image. On many occasions however, the result is that the client clams up, feels intimidated and remote from the vet and, with luck, will end up asking the nurse or the receptionist to repeat "the vet´s explanation".

11 Summarise key information for the client and ensure they have understood everything

The prestigious English veterinary consultant John Sheridan (www.veterinarybusinessbriefing.com) uses a methodology that shows to what extent client communication is a challenging task for many vets. The method consists of the following: over a period of three or four consecutive days, a questionnaire with three questions will be handed out after each appointment to both vets and clients for each to fill in (figure 4).

As the reader will probably guess, the vets had a great surprise when checking what their clients had understood...

Figure 4. Audit of Veterinary Communication Skills at the Practice.

Questions for the Vet

In this consultation that has just finished...

- **What has been the most important message that you gave the pet owner?**
- **What have you asked the pet owner to do from now on?**
- **When did you ask them to return to the practice with their pet?**

Questions for the Client

In this consultation that has just finished...

- **What has been the most important message that the vet has given you?**
- **What has the vet asked you to do from now on?**
- **When has the vet said that you should return with your pet to the veterinary practice?**

An effective technique to minimise this problem is to summarise the most important points at the end of each consultation:

- What have we found out?
- What does the veterinary practice have to do from now on?
- What should the pet owner do from now on?
- When should the patient return to the practice?

Also, it is advisable to close the conversation with the pet owner with a twofold question:

- "Mr. Jones, have we made everything clear? Would you like us to go over any of the information again?"

These two questions will clear up many misunderstandings, avoid clients calling with queries and will significantly improve compliance and ability to follow our health recommendations.

Nurturing the relationship: the follow-up after the consultation

It is not uncommon to find veterinary practices that lose between 20 and 40% of their patients from one year to the next. This means a real "hemorrhaging" for any business and severely limits growth potential, putting even its very survival at risk.

What are the most common causes of patient (client) loss for a veterinary practice?

Figure 5 ranks these causes according to the ability of the practice to influence them with their management systems:

Figure 5. Reasons for client loss.

Reasons outside the practice's control

- **Patient deaths (between 8 and 12% annually).**
- **Clients moving house (change of address) (1-2% annually).**
- **Losing a pet, donating it to someone else or to a rescue center (2-3% annually).**

Reasons within the practice's control

- **Customer dissatisfaction, resulting in an intentional change to another veterinary practice (from 2% to 5%).**
- **Lost clients due to poor communication by the practice (up to 20% annually!).**

Often many clients forget the date when they were supposed to return to the veterinary practice, and, as they are not actively contacted, they simply stop coming.

These figures are approximate and are based both on the author´s personal experience as a veterinary practice consultant and on several published studies[2].

The practices that have been concerned enough to ring those clients that had stopped coming to their veterinary practice for more than a year have discovered, to their surprise, that a significant percentage of them were not aware that they "were no longer clients".

Bearing this in mind, it is highly recommended that a **sequencial protocol for vaccination reminders** is routinely followed. The following procedure is recommended:

1. First letter (or email or text message to a mobile) 11 months after the last vaccination.
2. Second communication (by letter, email or text message to a mobile) to those clients who received the first communication a month ago and who have neither turned up at the practice or asked for an appointment.
3. Telephone call. For those clients who have also not responded to the second communication. This call ought to follow a structured protocol and always begin by showing interest and concern for the health of the pet. The purpose of the call must be to gather information about the status of the pet and, whenever possible, generate an appointment for its return to the veterinary practice.

Figure 6 shows an example of this type of telephone protocol:

Figure 6. Extract from a telephone protocol.

> "Good morning (afternoon), Mr/Mrs. (client name), my name is (name of the caller) and I´m calling from the ABC Veterinary Hospital.
>
> Following a review of our patient records we have realised that (name of the pet) has not been to the practice for the last 12 months and so we are calling, firstly to confirm that (name of pet) is well and secondly –just in case you had forgotten– to remind you that the last vaccination (name of the pet) had has already expired and unless it has been given again over the past 12 months..."

A thoughtful touch, surgical follow-up calls

Various studies have been carried out on the marketing activities of veterinary practices[3] and it has been discovered that one of the actions that had the most positive impact on clients was an unexpected call from the veterinary practice to find out how the pet was recovering after surgery.

The veterinary practice should establish a specific policy for these types of calls, clearly defining the following issues:

- For which kinds of procedures (it is suggested that they are limited to surgery).
- When (it is suggested they are made 48 hours after the surgery was done).
- What is said (show interest in the recovery of the patient and anticipate any possible concerns the owner might have, take advantage of the call to remind the owner of the date of the follow-up visit).

These calls can (and should) be made by non-veterinary practice staff. They provide an excellent public relations exercise that most clients do not expect and also help to identify and proactively resolve any possible concerns or worries. In the event that any of these calls result in concerns of a medical nature that require discussion with a vet, the person in charge of making the calls will take the responsibility to gather together all the relevant information and call the client back. It is advisable to create a monitoring report where the person in charge of making the calls systematically records the calls made, the calls to be made, the comments received from clients and any action required.

Telephone services: closing the circle

Now we will discuss some key concepts around telephone services at the veterinary practice.

Professional, standardised greeting

"ABC Veterinary Practice, good morning, Charles speaking. How can I help you?" If the phone is ringing non-stop and we have no time to make a full greeting, the following points are considered essential: "ABC Veterinary Practice, how can I help you?".

Filtering and returning calls for vets

When the client wants to talk to a vet at the practice, the person answering the telephone ought to try to obtain the following information:

- Name of the client / patient.
- Time of the call.
- Reason for the call.

The first option should be to try to directly resolve the owner´s concern without passing them to a vet. If this is not possible and the vet is not available, the client will be given the option of being called back by the practice at some point during the day.

Questions about price made over the telephone

The recommended protocol in these situations is as follows:

1. Ask the caller if they are already a client at the practice. This will help us to decide which information to provide.

2. If the person who calls us is not a client, ask for their name and address so that they can be sent written information about our practice (a practice leaflet). In this way we can make sure that the caller is informed about our services and it also helps to deter possible "information hunters" or informers for the competition.

3 For those specific services that we have agreed we can give prices for over the telephone (normally routine procedures like consultations, vaccinations, prophylactic dental treatments, spaying, etc.), always explain the value of the service first and then give the price. The following example illustrates the way to manage these calls:

Example

Question:
–"How much does a booster vaccine for a dog cost at your practice?"

Answer:

VALUE ➡ –"In our practice the vaccinations are always given following a full 15 minute physical examination by a vet. During this examination the sight, ears, joints, weight, temperature, heart rate and urogenital system of the pet are all checked". "Once the examination has been completed, and providing the patient is in good health, the vaccination will be given".

PRICE ➡ "The price of this service is 34 monetary units".

Notice how this way of answering conveys to the client two very distinct pieces of information: the price, and the value that the client gets in return for that price. This represents a significant departure from the standard procedures of many practices that only give out the price of services without explaining what they consist of. The practice in our example has a greater probability of being chosen by the client. Even if the client decides to call a second practice for comparison, we can imagine what will happen if at the second practice they are given only information on price (for example "24 euros") and nothing about the value of the service. Is it not reasonable to assume that the client will doubt the quality of the service at the second practice? Probably they will be asking themselves if at the second (cheaper) practice the physical examination lasts for 15 minutes, or if it will be done by a vet, or if it will be as comprehensive as the first practice...

Phrases to avoid when using the telephone[4]

There are a number of phrases that those of us who frequently call veterinary practices hear more often than we would like. Now we will review some of these expressions and see why they are incorrect.

"Sorry, Dr. White still has not returned from lunch"
We are giving out unnecessary information (the lunchtimes of the vet are irrelevant) and the word "still" suggests delay, that the vet is taking an excessively long lunch break...

"Just now I don't know where the vet is, can I take your number and ask them to call you back later?"
The second part of the phrase is perfect (orientated towards the client) but the first part conveys the feeling of a lack of internal organization and poor communication within the practice team. It would be sufficient to say, "The vet is not here at the moment, may I have your number? I will make sure we call you when he returns".

"I think the vet is having breakfast. Don't worry, when she returns I will tell her that you called"
Yet again, the first part of this phrase combines the mistakes of the first and second responses.

"Right now the vet is really busy, she has had a terrible morning. Would you mind leaving a message?"
This response conveys an image of internal chaos, that the practice (and the vet) is overwhelmed by events and there is a lack of management control.

"The vet is at the dentist, he will be back this afternoon"
This information is not relevant to the client. It conveys the impression that staff at the practice are absent for personal reasons during working hours, when that is not necessarily the case.

"Today he has gone home early"
This information is irrelevant to the pet owner. It can convey an unprofessional image, a lack of internal discipline, etc.

"The vet should be back next Monday".
Here the use of the modal verb "should" carries negative overtones. It seems as if things are not very clear at this practice, as if there was a certain lack of management control.

"Well, in principle the invoice is correct".
This is not the most reassuring way to tell a client that their invoice is correct.

"It looks like we have calculated the estimate correctly".
Would we like to hear from our mechanic "it looks like the brake is fixed now"?

"Best if you call back later rather than have to wait for the vet to call you back".
No comment!

"Sorry for the delay, the phones have been ringing non-stop".
Yet again, there is a feeling of helplessness and a failure on the part of the business to provide adequate resources.

"I don't understand why someone didn't call you earlier to explain".
Here it appears as if the person answering the telephone does not work at the practice. It seems as if the problem was actually nothing to do with them but rather a third party (the business) from whom they distance themselves in order not to appear responsible in front of the client. This type of response generates confusion and deep mistrust in the client.

Key Chapter Concepts

- We must make sure that all the "non-clinical" elements that make up a part of a client's visit to our practice (telephone calls, reception, staff they have dealings with, the appearance of the facilities) result in a pleasant experience.

- The best way to prepare for a consultation is to start working before the client arrives at our practice. To this end, it is essential that the appointment book is organised with a system of scheduled appointments and the medical records are reviewed in order to identify any outstanding health issues that need attention.

- The main reason for losing customers is poor communication from the veterinary practice's side. We must refine our protocols for monitoring booster reminders and establish a call system to recover lost clients.

- As with medical procedures, we should create client care protocols for our consultations. We must clearly define what we say and how we say it.

- The telephone is not just an instrument for receiving annoying calls from clients that stop us from working...
  If well used, the telephone can be the main tool to sell our services and a resource for client retention and loyalty.

References

1. Ettinger, S. *Textbook of Veterinary Internal Medicine*, 6th ed. Saunders, 2004.
2. AVEPA - Hill's Pet Nutrition. Estudio de Cumplimiento (Compliance Study), 2006.
3. Opperman, M. *The Art of Veterinary Practice Management.* Veterinary Medicine Publishing Group, 1999.
4. Adapted from Finch, Ll. Telephone Courtesy and Client Service. American Veterinary Medical Association (www.avma.org), 1999.

Surveys
Listening to the voice of the client

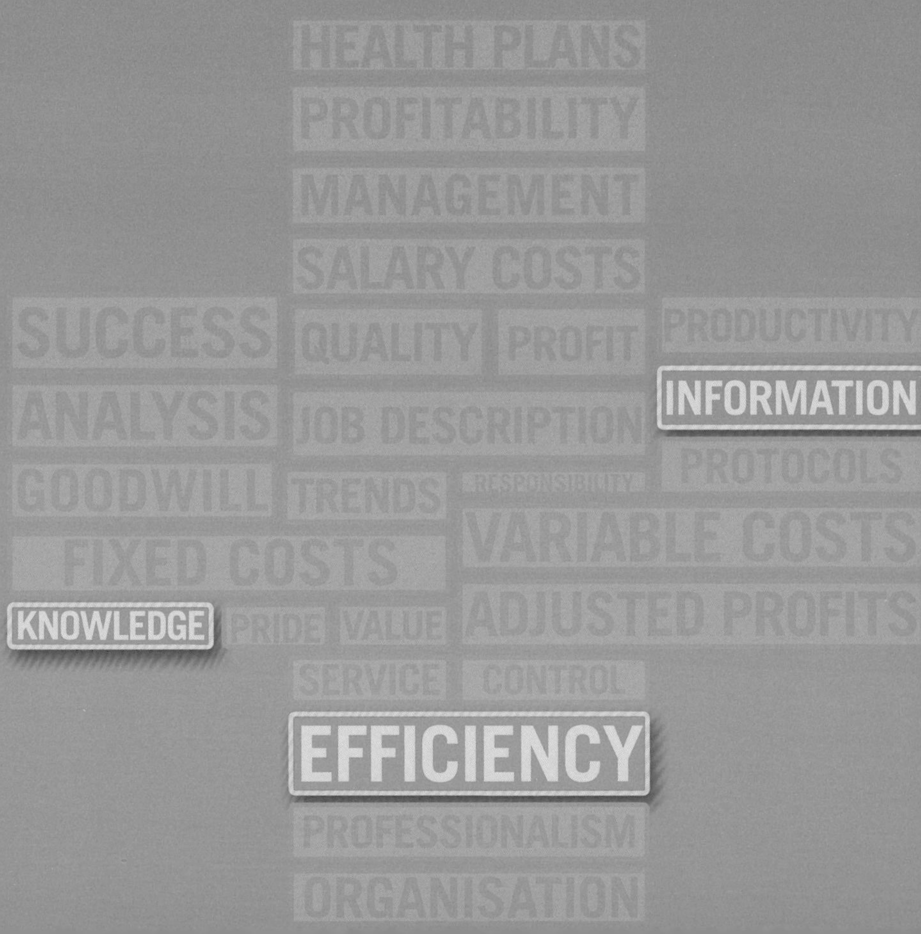

8

It is recommended that client surveys are carried out as they provide the following benefits for a veterinary practice:

- **To obtain relevant information to aid the decision-making process**
  Most surveys are carried out for this reason. To find out how our clients found out about us, to know how they rate our telephone service, to find out which other veterinary practices they have been to apart from ours, to check which of our services they are aware, or unaware, of...These are just a few examples of the many questions that we can study through surveys.

- **To motivate and evaluate staff**
  According to the saying that is popular amongst managers "if it is measured, it will be done". Just the fact that our staff are aware that clients are rating our service can be a great additional motivator. On the other hand, the information obtained from these surveys can become valuable criteria for assessing the performance of our staff. It is increasingly common to find practices where a variable part of the vets' remuneration is linked to the results of client satisfaction surveys.

- **To enhance the image of the veterinary practice**
  Just the fact of carrying out these surveys sends a clear message from the veterinary practice management to both clients and their own employees at the practice. They show that management concern for customer satisfaction is not just a lot of hot air but it actually translates into specific initiatives for which practice resources are used.

What is the best way to carry out client surveys?

The vet that is considering carrying out a client survey is often confronted with a number of questions about the methodology to follow: Is it better to do the survey by telephone, or by post? Is it better to do it yourself or hire an external agency to do it? What is the minimum number of clients that should be surveyed to ensure we can draw reliable conclusions? Should the surveys be anonymous or should the client identify themselves? Is it advisable to share the results with our team, even if they are negative?

It is almost impossible to provide a definitive answer to these questions that will be equally applicable to all situations. However, certain decision-making criteria can be applied:

Telephone, post or neither of them?

The main advantages of the telephone over the post are speed, the interactivity (you can engage in a dialogue with the client) and a higher response rate. On the other hand, the telephone has the inconvenience of being more intrusive, and some clients can become annoyed at being contacted at certain times of the day when they are busy or by the length of the survey. With respect to cost, although the telephone might seem more economical (as long as we call from the practice and only to landlines), the cost of the person's time that is making the calls must also be taken into account.

An alternative option that works well in many veterinary practices is to ask the client to fill in an exit survey at the practice that can be put into a mailbox or a "ballot box" designed specifically for that purpose. In this way we can combine economy (as we are not incurring postage or telephone charges) with speed and a high response rate. Most clients will be happy to spend between 3 and 5 minutes answering a survey, particularly if the receptionists are properly trained to offer it proactively. It might be a nice gesture to offer a little something to the pet (for example a healthy treat) to keep it busy while the owner fills in the questionnaire.

Should you create a survey "in-house" or contract an external agency?

In this author's experience there are advantages to doing the survey yourself and using someone on the team, especially if you opt for a telephone survey. This is because of the easy access to patient clinical records, because you know the clients better and because you can take advantage of the calls to resolve client concerns as well as arrange new appointments. The client will probably also see this familiar contact as a genuine expression of your concern towards them rather than if the call was received from a call centre. However, in order to make the calls from the practice, it is essential to arrange for a second line to be installed (otherwise you run the risk of blocking incoming calls) and also to allocate a specific time for someone on the team to make them. If these requirements cannot be met, then it is better to consider the option of using an external agency or opt for either postal surveys or printed surveys for use in the practice.

What is the minimum number of clients that we should survey?

Without going into any technical detail about statistics, it is recommended as a rule of thumb that a minimum of 75 surveys are carried out in order to obtain some reliable information. This figure should be adjusted according to the characteristics of the practice and, above all, to the degree of detail desired once the data has been analysed. If, for example, we want to analyse the differences between four vets at the same practice with respect to client satisfaction, it is recommended that 300 (4 x 75) surveys are carried out. However, if we only want to assess the overall level of client satisfaction with the practice, it would be enough to carry out a survey of 75 clients.

Is it a good idea to share the survey results with our team?

It is highly advisable to do so. It motivates the team and helps them to have a better understanding of the clients' point of view regarding the practice. In the case of a negative result, the correct thing would be to discuss the reasons for it with the team and involve them in the search for possible solutions. If the negative result is clearly linked to a particular member of staff, then the most sensible and effective thing to do would often be to speak to them in private.

Practical examples of survey formats

Now let's see three survey examples with clearly different formats and objectives.

1. Client satisfaction survey[1]

Some interesting aspects of this survey format are:

- **Scale**. Note how an even number of ranges (four evaluation grades to choose from) avoids replies that "sit on the fence" and force the client to at least discriminate between a "poor" or "good" level of service.
- **Coding**. The section to be completed by the practice at the top of the questionnaire will give us the option to separately analyse the results by vet or by nurse employed.
- **Prediction of client's future intention.** The most important question of all those on the survey is the last one, as it condenses the client's overall evaluation of the practice into just one question. With their reply to this question the client will be able to tell us if the value that they have received from our service exceeds the price they have paid and thereby indicates if they had a positive experience. This is an indirect way to ask about our prices, an issue that it would not be appropriate to ask clients directly as the responses would be skewed by definition (no-one in their right mind is going to tell us we are cheap and then be faced with the prospect of us raising our prices...).

Note ➡ If we want to obtain an honest answer, it is important to keep this kind of survey anonymous and confidential as we are asking the client to value our service. For that we must ensure the clients can fill in the questionnaire in private and they can put the survey themselves in a mailbox or "ballot box" designed for that purpose.

Please help us to improve our client care and the quality of our services. Your opinion is very important to us.			
Is this the 1st time you have visited our practice?	YES / NO	Vet:....................................	Survey nº:..........................
Have you come with an emergency?	YES / NO	Nurse:..	
(Section to be completed by the practice)		Pet DOG/CAT/...	

Please circle the number that best describes the experience you have had with us today	Very poor	Poor	Good	Excellent
A. Telephone Service				
1. We answered your call quickly	1	2	3	4
2. Courteous and efficient receptionist	1	2	3	4
3. Your questions were answered clearly	1	2	3	4
B. Our Reception/waiting room				
1. Our staff were friendly and efficient	1	2	3	4
2. Your waiting time was reasonable	1	2	3	4
3. Your questions were answered clearly	1	2	3	4
4. You were comfortable and well looked after while you were waiting	1	2	3	4
C. Our Facilities				
1. It was easy to get here	1	2	3	4
2. The entrance was well signposted	1	2	3	4
3. The hospital was very clean	1	2	3	4
4. There were no unpleasant smells	1	2	3	4
5. There was interesting reading material in reception	1	2	3	4
6. Cleanliness and tidiness of the consulting room	1	2	3	4
D. Our nurses				
1. The professionalism of our nurses	1	2	3	4
2. My pet and I were well looked after	1	2	3	4
E. Our Vets				
1. The vet gave you enough time	1	2	3	4
2. The vet explained everything that they were doing well	1	2	3	4
3. Your questions were well answered	1	2	3	4
4. How thorough was the physical examination of your pet?	1	2	3	4
5. My pet and I were well looked after	1	2	3	4
F. Services and opening times				
1. Type and variety of clinical services	1	2	3	4
2. Normal opening hours convenient	1	2	3	4
How would you rate our overall service?	1	2	3	4
The next time you have to go to the vet, would you use us again?	YES / NO	Why? (if the answer is no)		

Please use the box below to make any suggestions or observations.

2. Survey to get to know more about our clients

Circle the correct answer	
1. How did you find us?	
Saw it when passing	x
Recommended by someone else	x
Yellow pages	x
Internet	x
Referred by another vet	x
2. Have you been to another veterinary practice?	
No	x
Yes	x
Which one?	
3. How do you normally get here?	
Walking	x
By car	x
On public transport	x
4. How often do you connect to the internet?	
Never	x
Almost never	x
From time to time	x
Daily	x
5. Indicate which of the following services you think we offer	
Vaccinations	x
Surgery	x
Blood tests	x
X rays	x
Behavioural advice	x
Groomer	x
Nutricional advice	x
Wormers and flea control	x
Physiotherapy	x

The advantage of this type of survey lies in the fact that the questions devised are not of a sensitive nature, that is to say the client will not normally have any qualms about answering them directly. This will allow our reception team to be proactive in handing them out to clients rather than leaving a pile of them lying around on the desk unnoticed by clients.

Question 1 will allow us to better understand how important the different ways of reaching new clients are, which will put us in a better position to consider our investment in some of the published advertising media such as Yellow Pages.

Question 2 's objective is to let us know which practices our clients compare us with and therefore the expected standard which we must measure ourselves against.

Question 3 can help us to better assess how important it is to our clients that we offer parking facilities (for example making arrangements with a local car park).

Question 4 will provide guidance on the convenience of using digital media to communicate with our clients (web page, emails, e-newsletters…).

Finally, **question 5** has the function of making us angry and complain bitterly at the low level of knowledge that our clients have about our services. Usually this is due to a lack of effort on our part to communicate it properly.

3. Surveys which are amusing and generate PR for our practice[2]

This survey, adapted from an extended model developed by the AAHA (American Animal Hospital Association), can be an excellent PR tool for our practice. Just imagine the smiles of the clients when they receive a newsletter with the result highlights from the questionnaire, or consider the psychological effect that it could have on the employees knowing the extent to which the clients are emotionally attached to their pets or even visualise the attention-grabbing headlines that the local media (press or radio) would be willing to print or broadcast if you let them have a short press release with the results from your practice.

If you were on a desert island and you could only take one companion, which of the following would you take?

- ☐ Another person
- ☐ A dog
- ☐ A cat
- ☐ No one

Have you ever taken your pet on holiday with you?

- ☐ Yes
- ☐ No

Do you think that your pet has any human personality traits?

- ☐ They are stubborn
- ☐ They are lazy
- ☐ They have feelings
- ☐ They are inquisitive
- ☐ They rather fancy themselves
- ☐ None of the above

What is the likelihood that you would risk your life – should it be necessary –for your pet?

- ☐ Very probably
- ☐ Quite likely
- ☐ Under no circumstances

Who is the best listener?

- ☐ Your best friend
- ☐ Your partner
- ☐ Someone else in the family
- ☐ Your pet

How often do you think about your pet when you are away from them during the day?

- ☐ At least once a day
- ☐ Several times a day
- ☐ Every hour
- ☐ All the time
- ☐ Almost never

Does your pet like to watch TV?

- ☐ Yes
- ☐ No

Where does your pet sleep?

- ☐ Outside the house
- ☐ In a room of the house
- ☐ Sometimes in my bed
- ☐ Always in my bed

Have you ever got a pet to keep another pet company?

- ☐ Yes
- ☐ No

Some practical considerations relating to surveys

- **Invest time in its design.** It is essential that the questions are clear and precise. Ask family and friends for help to read and test a draft before distributing the final version among clients.

- **Design closed questions that are easier to put in a table.** Whenever possible we should favour closed questions, that is to say those with just the two answers of "yes/no" or at least a menu of set responses. This will greatly facilitate the analysis and presentation of the results.

- **Use the results of the surveys in a constructive way.** If we use them to single out or punish people on our team, we will generate such great resentment and internal resistance to this tool that it will be difficult to get anyone to help us do them in future.

Focus groups, in-depth interviews and other qualitative research techniques

The quantitative surveys we have seen up to now are not the only means of obtaining information from clients at a veterinary practice's disposal. On occasion, when it is of interest to analyse issues of a more qualitative nature, such as our clients' deepest motivations or their attitude towards us, we need to use other kinds of techniques.

A methodology commonly used by companies in other sectors is what is known as focus groups. They aim to bring together a group of clients (or potential clients) and encourage them to talk along the lines of a structured script under the supervision of a moderator. Another related technique is the in-depth interview, where an interviewer raises a series of questions to which the client responds in detail.

The difference with the quantitative surveys is that the qualitative techniques do not allow us to extrapolate their results to the whole of our clientele, however they do have the important advantage that they enable us to gain access to a richer and deeper level of information. Given their greater complexity, the use of specialised professionals is recommended to carry them out and interpret the results obtained.

Key Chapter Concepts

- Surveys are a good tool to get to know our clients better, to motivate our staff and to secure a good business image.
- To carry out in-house surveys using our own staff is often an option worth considering.
- We can use the surveys in order to discover the perception that our clients have of us, to get to know more about them and even to obtain good publicity for our practice.
- Surveys are not useful for obtaining all types of information. More sophisticated methodologies exist (like focus groups or in-depth interviews) that give us access to much deeper levels of information about our clients.

References

1. Format developed from the original by Gerald Snyder (www.vethelp.us) and adapted with suggestions from students of the Master of Administration and Management of Veterinary Practices from AVEPA-UAB.
2. Format developed from the original by AAHA (www.aahanet.org) and adapted with suggestions from students of the Master of Administration and Management of Veterinary Practices from AVEPA-UAB.

Preventative medicine versus palliative medicine: **a paradigm shift**

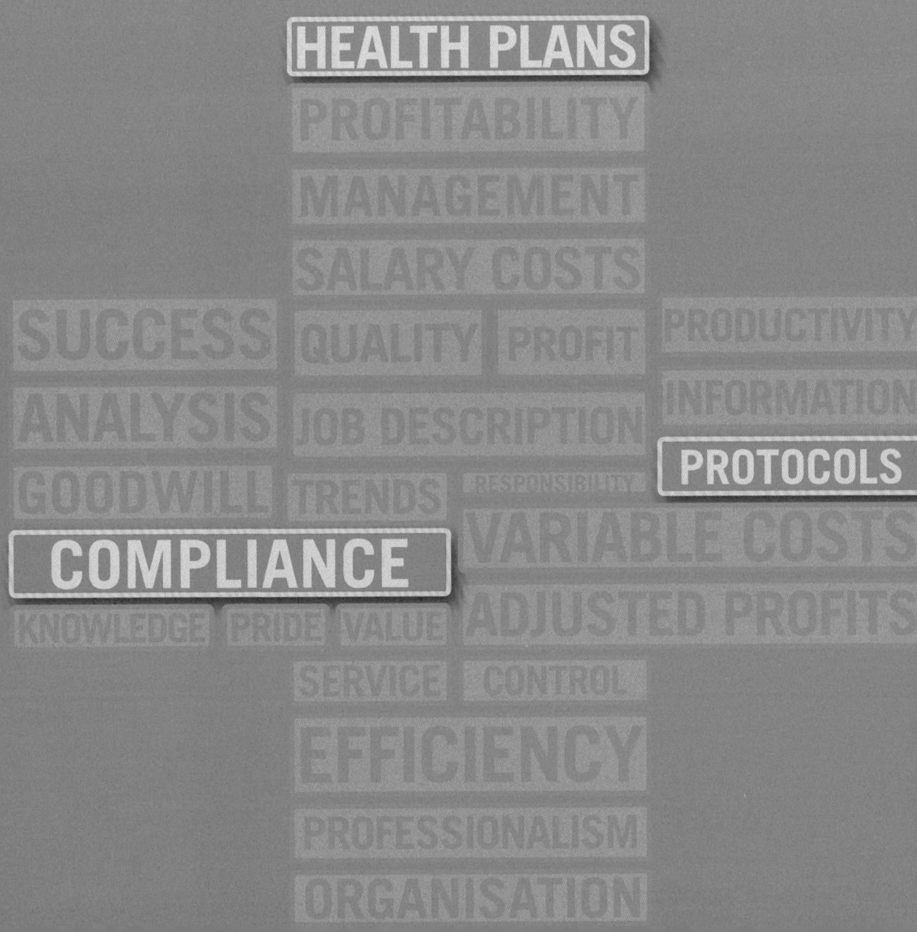

9

Preventive medicine is the medicine of the future for most vets. Increasingly, pets will not visit veterinary practices **when they are sick**, but in order **not to get sick**. This change of approach, which should be led by vets themselves, will be a real revolution in the way we work and understand the profession.

Veterinary practice turnover =
Number of active patients x Average frequency of visits x Average income per visit

If we consider this veterinary practice turnover model, we will see that one of the three factors (the number of active patients) will be unlikely to grow much in the coming years. Socio-demographic trends (increase in lone households, increase in the number of professional couples without children and with busy schedules, the rising cost of living space, tax burdens and local government regulations on pet owners) do not augur well for a significant rise in domestic pet ownership. In fact, in recent years we have already seen a clear tendency towards the gradual replacement of large breed dogs for medium-sized or small dogs, cats or so-called "exotics" (reptiles, rabbits, hamsters). Presumably in the future therefore, income growth for many veterinary practices will have to come from the other two factors in the equation: average frequency of visits and average income per visit. Preventative medicine can play a key role in both.

Another underlying trend in our sector is the gradual evolution toward specialisation. This is a reflection of what is happening in human medicine. The speed and complexity of the technical disciplines make it almost impossible for anyone to be an expert in more than one animal species or in several physiological systems... Hence the rise in the number of qualified specialists and referral centres. Just as is happening now in the United States, the day will come when it will be the pet owners themselves who will demand, on their own initiative, the services of veterinary specialists. These specialists will provide their services in large referral hospitals or in specialist centres that will receive sufficient cases to make their exclusive dedication viable. The appearance of this kind of large centre, with significant investment in equipment and highly qualified staff, will be a major challenge to the local, more traditional first opinion practice. As happens in any sector of economic activity, whoever wants to succeed will have to find their niche in the market. This author predicts that those local first opinion practices that will adapt best to this revolution in the market will be those that specialise in preventative medicine and offer a personalised service to clients in the vicinity.

The starting point: the current situation

The term compliance is used to describe the situation in which a patient is receiving the level of medical care that its vet considers to be the optimal. In all the main studies to date[1,2], it has been shown that, despite what many vets think, the majority of patients in veterinary practices receive health care that is far from **optimal.** Vets tend to overestimate the levels of compliance in their patients, probably because they do not use rigorous quantitative measures to analyse this issue.

In these studies, it was considered that a patient was **in compliance** with the different areas of health if it met the following requirements (fig. 1):

Figure 1. Compliance criteria for the main areas of health in preventative medicine.

Leishmania/Philaria (in areas where is it endemic)	That the patient has received the preventative treatment following the protocol advised by the vet and has had any diagnostic tests as and when the vet recommended it.
Preventative dental treatments	That the patient has received prophylactic dental treatments if their dental condition score is in the range 2, 3 or 4.
Prescription diets	If the patient suffers from renal disease, urolithiasis or FLUTD, chronic or acute gastrointestinal disorders or obesity that it will be regularly fed on the appropriate prescription diet.
Geriatric profile	That if the patient is an older pet it has had a blood and urine test at least once a year.
Vaccinations	That the patient must be vaccinated following the protocol advised by its vet and at least against distemper, hepatitis, leptospirosis, parainfluenza and parvovirus (for dogs), and rhinotracheitis, calicivirus and panleukopenia (for cats).
Pre-anaesthetic profile	That if the patient has undergone surgery, it had all the pre-anaesthetic tests recommended by the practice.

Some of the main conclusions of these studies were as follows:

1. Only a very small number of vets regularly monitored these indicators and therefore the majority were not rigorously measuring the percentage of their canine and feline patients that were in compliance with each health area.

2. In the vast majority of practices analysed, documented levels of patient compliance were significantly lower than what the vets had estimated before the start of the study.

3. When the clinical histories were examined, it was found that the main documented reason for compliance failure in all areas of health was not the refusal by pet owners to follow the vet's recommendations. There were many failures of compliance due to inadequate protocols (e.g. failure to request pre-anaesthetic profiles for risk patients, or failure to record the dental condition of all patients during each physical examination), an absence of recommendations or inadequate patient follow up (especially in treatment of chronic conditions).

4. Besides the obvious negative effect of these low levels of compliance on the pet's health, there was an important financial implication. It was estimated that the average North American veterinary clinic would increase its annual turnover by more than 132,000 dollars if they were able to raise compliance rates by 10% among patients in all the areas of health analysed. This finding was consistent with the results of the analysis done in Europe (Spain), where it was estimated that the financial impact of this improvement would be in the region of 100,000 euros a year.

The five key points of preventative medicine

In order for a veterinary practice to make significant progress in their shifting focus towards preventative medicine, the following requirements must be met:

1 Conviction

It is very difficult for a professional to recommend with any conviction a service they do not believe in. The first thing we have to do is openly and honestly discuss with our veterinary team what the practice's philosophy is regarding preventative medicine. What is the standard of preventative medicine we would wish for our own pets? In all conscience we ought to recommend the same level of medical care (no more, no less) than we would want for our own pets. If we are not truly convinced of the benefits of preventative medicine, then it is better to be realistic and focus our efforts elsewhere.

2 Obsession with keeping thorough clinical records of each patient

The medical history is an essential tool for good clinical management of the patient and good financial management of the client. It is an important document with medical, legal and financial implications. An incomplete medical history, where no health recommendations have been recorded as being refused by a client, can be decisive in the negative resolution of a legal dispute. In the United States, expert valuers of veterinary practices put lower valuations on practices with badly documented medical histories.

If it is not measured, it won't get done. Similarly what is not written down, is hardly going to be measured. Therefore it is essential that our team is aware of the need to write these records professionally. A good medical history ought to at least contain the following information for each consultation with a patient:

- Reason for the consultation.
- Detailed information provided by the owner.
- Detailed findings from the physical examination (including weight, temperature, physical and dental condition as well as a detailed list of the symptoms).

- Diagnostic tests proposed, carried out and / or rejected by the client.
- Diagnosis (whenever possible) or assessment of the patient.
- Treatment options presented to the client.
- Treatment option chosen.
- Outcome of treatment (when the information is available).
- The vet and the nurse that were involved.
- Monitoring system used in this case (according to the system of the 3 R´s explained previously: re-call, re-check, re-minder).

It is also advisable that nursing or reception staff review the following questions with the pet owner at least once a year:

- Confirm their postal address, home and mobile telephone numbers and email address.
- Ask if they have any travel plans in the near future (in case they have relevant implications for the pet's health).
- Confirm the status of vaccinations and wormers/flea control for the pet.
- Record the type of food that the pet is fed.
- For adult and older pets, check to see whether there has been any change in ability to tolerate exercise, if a lump or spot has appeared recently, or if the owner has detected any significant change in behaviour.

These questions will help to gather relevant information from a medical standpoint, they will convey a sense of professionalism to the client and in addition will help to educate pet owners without the need to "sell" them anything.

3 Educate, don't sell

Educated clients are those **who buy** services, there is no need to sell them anything... We must redefine the role of the veterinary practice as a place where clients are educated so they can enjoy the best possible relationship with their pets. We live in an information society, where clients come to our practice after having read on the Internet information of varying quality about the health of their pet... Eagerness and demand for information is now greater than ever from our clients. Bearing this in mind we must be prepared to lead this process, because if we do not then our clients will find other sources of information and probably not asact accordingly if we do not then our clients will find other sources of information and probably not as reliable. If we really agree with this philosophy, then we must begin to act accordingly:

- We must select and appraise our vets taking into account their communication skills with clients.
- We must facilitate this educational process by providing our team with the appropriate resources: written information for clients, visual aids in the consulting rooms (posters, atlases, anatomical models).
- We must invest time and energy in explaining things to clients: our estimates, our treatment plans and even our invoices must aim to educate clients.
- We must encourage those activities and programmes that follow this line: newsletters, puppy classes, staff training in communication skills, etc.

4 Create protocols for preventative medicine

What is unjustifiable and indefensible before a client is that their pet receives a different level of physical examination, or different diagnostic tests or a different treatment recommendation depending on which vet in our practice they have seen.

- Should we, or should we not, record the dental condition of all patients during each consultation? What specific recommendations do we give the client depending on the dental condition score of their pet?
- Should we, or should we not, record the body condition of all patients during each consultation? What specific recommendations should we make to the client depending on the body condition score of their pet?
- Do we, or do we not, recommend neutering of young dogs and cats? At what age do we recommend this procedure? Do we note in the medical record if the recommendation was made and the owner's response? How do we make this recommendation to the client? Do we have a fact sheet about it?
- Do we have a protocol for the early detection of joint problems in risk patients? Have we defined how to carry out a physical examination specifically for this type of condition and when to do it?
- What is our policy with respect to pre-anaesthetic profiles? Are we going to **offer** them or simply inform clients that these profiles are an inherent part of the surgical procedure and we routinely include them in all our estimates?
- What about the blood and urine tests for older patients?

All these questions deserve to be discussed internally and a common standpoint should be agreed (in writing) by each veterinary practice.

5 Measure

If we indoctrinate our team with the importance of preventative medicine but then they never see us monitoring it or measuring progress, we will be sending a message that lacks credibility.

It is not enough just to implement the protocols discussed in the previous section, we must also check their use. We must check a sample of medical records and treatment plans prepared by our vets at regular intervals.

Practical application: Puppy health plan

Detailed below is an example of a preventative medicine programme for puppies[3]. What is important in this example is not so much its contents as its **working method.**

First: define the health standard

The first step is to define, together with our veterinary team, what standard of health we want to offer our patients (figure 2). How would we like to look after these patients?

Second: practise what you preach

If we are serious and convinced that this is the optimal health standard for our patients, then we should also apply it to our own pets. The best way for our team of vets and support staff to talk with conviction to clients about the benefits of a service is for them to use it on their own pets. A practical way to achieve this is for our employees to have access to these programmes for their pet under very favourable conditions, as part of their overall remuneration package.

Figure 2. Puppy Health Plan.

1st visit (before 6 weeks)	
Thorough physical examination. Purchase valuation (where applicable). Faecal analysis. Wormers. Flea/tick control. Protection against leishmania.	Explanations: • Diet advice. • Behaviour advice*. • Home health care (i.e. brushing teeth, grooming, nail clipping, ears). • Review of the reminders system. • Review health plan. * offer specific session(s).
2nd visit (at 6 weeks)	
Thorough physical examination. Puppy vaccination*. Protection against leishmania.	Explanations: • Review of worming/flea control guidelines. • Review health plan.
3rd visit (at 9 weeks)	
Thorough physical examination. Quadrivalent vaccination*. Home dental care.	Explanations: • Review health plan.
4th visit (at 13 weeks)	
Thorough physical examination. Vaccination (booster). Microchip.	Explanations: • Review of worming/flea control guidelines. • Review health plan.
5th visit (at 6 months)	
Thorough physical examination. Rabies vaccine*. Pre-anaesthetic profile. Examine and photograph dental condition. Photograph/video of joint function.	Explanations: • Review of worming/flea control guidelines. • Diet review (change of calorie intake). • Reproductive health and neutering. • Review adult health plan.

* Vaccination protocols to be adjusted on a country basis.

Prepare information for our clients, emphasising value

Once the content of the service has been designed, we must explain it in a way that is both clear and attractive to clients. The key is to communicate the advantages or benefits the service brings, both to them and their pets. Many times we are so obsessed with explaining the technical features of a veterinary service that we forget to tell the client about its value to their pet. Figure 3 shows a puppy health plan, highlighting its many benefits for the client and the patient.

Figure 3. Puppy Health Plan: information for the owner.

What does the puppy health programme at ABC Veterinary Hospital consist of?

The first year of a pet's life is the most important in relation to its health and quality of life. Things such as good immune protection, proper socialisation and behaviour management, good feeding habits, physical exercise, etc. will be established during this period. ABC Veterinary Hospital, which has 20 years experience of caring for pets, recommends that during the first year the following advice is followed:

First check-up (before 6 weeks old)	
Procedure	**Purpose / Explanation**
Thorough physical examination.	To check eyes, ears, urogenital tracts, anal glands, weight and diet, behaviour, skin and coat.
Faecal analysis.	To detect the presence of intestinal parasites.
Worming.	To protect against intestinal parasites.
Flea / tick control.	To protect against parasites of the skin and coat.
Protection against leishmaniasis.	To prevent this serious disease being transmitted by mosquito bites.
Information for the owner (review of the main dietary issues, exercise, home health care, behaviour and socialisation).	For optimal care of the puppy at home.
Second check-up (at 6 weeks old)	
Procedure	**Purpose / Explanation**
Detailed physical examination.	To check eyes, ears, urogenital tracts, anal glands, weight and diet, behaviour, skin and coat.
Vaccine protection (puppy vaccine)*.	To boost their immunity against the main potentially life threatening diseases.
Worming.	To protect against intestinal parasites.
Flea / tick control.	To protect against parasites of the skin and coat.
Third check-up (at 9 weeks old)	
Procedure	**Purpose / Explanation**
Detailed physical examination.	To check eyes, ears, urogenital tracts, anal glands, weight and diet, behaviour, skin and coat.
Vaccine protection (tetravalent vaccine) *.	To boost their immunity against the main potentially life threatening diseases.
Introduction to home dental care.	To educate the puppy in healthy habits.

* Vaccination protocols to be adjusted on a country basis.

Fourth check-up (at 13 weeks old)	
Procedure	**Purpose / Explanation**
Thorough physical examination.	To check eyes, ears, urogenital tracts, anal glands, weight and diet, behaviour, skin and coat.
Vaccine protection (tetravalent vaccine) *.	To boost their immunity against the main potentially life threatening diseases.
Worming.	To protect against intestinal parasites.
Flea / tick control.	To protect against parasites of the skin and coat.
Microchip (where applicable).	A legal obligation. It will help with identification and recovery of the pet if it gets lost or escapes.
Fifth check-up (at 6 months old)	
Procedure	**Purpose / Explanation**
Thorough physical examination.	To check eyes, ears, urogenital tracts, anal glands, weight and diet, behaviour, skin and coat.
Vaccine protection (rabies) *.	To boost their immunity against the main potentially life threatening diseases.
Worming.	To protect against intestinal parasites.
Flea / tick control.	To protect against parasites of the skin and coat.
Pre-anaesthetic profile.	To know in advance the best method of anaesthesia for future surgical interventions.
Diet review.	Switch to an adult diet (lower in calories) to avoid weight problems.
Photographic study of dental condition.	For early detection of gum or tooth problems.
Joint health study (video).	For early detection of joint and /or mobility problems.
Information for the owner.	Reproductive health. Advantages of neutering. Available alternatives.

* Vaccination protocols to be adjusted on a country basis.

Design a control and monitoring system for the team to use

If we are not willing to monitor and measure the results of the programme, it is better that we do not start it. Better a single health plan that has been fairly well designed and superbly executed than five that have been brilliantly designed and poorly implemented. Figure 4 shows an example of a monitoring template for one of these programmes.

Figure 4. Puppy Health Plan: monitoring template.

Patient: **Lucas**
Record nº: **7267**

1st visit (before 6 weeks old)	Vet/ Auxiliar	Answer from the owner	Action to be taken by the practice	Record date
Thorough physical examination.	Charles	Done.	Create reminder in computer.	(at 6 weeks).
Post-purchase valuation (where applicable).	Charles	Done.		
Faecal sample.	Charles	Requested appointment so it can be done another day.	Schedule another appointment.	(15 days later).
Wormer.	Charles	Done.	Create reminder in computer.	(at 6 weeks).
Flea/tick control.	Charles	Done.	Create reminder in computer.	(at 6 weeks).
Protection against leishmania.	Charles	Decision postponed.	Remind at next consultation.	
Explanations	**Louise**			
Diet advice.	Louise	Done.		
Behaviour advice.	Louise	Not offered, still outstanding.		
Home health care.	Louise	Done.		
Review reminder system.	Louise	Done.		
Review health plan.	Louise	Done.		

The fact that our computer software does not have a template like this is no excuse for failing to monitor properly. We can start by doing a draft on paper, or alternatively develop it ourselves using one of the standard software applications on the computer. Once the programme has been fully tested and fine tuned, we can ask our software provider (if necessary) to develop an application for us that is useful not only for this health plan but also for others (kittens, adults, older pets). Remember that IT is only a tool that enables us to carry out our work, and as such should not dictate what we do, or do not do, in our veterinary practice. If we have clear ideas about our business, computer-based tools can be created to accommodate our ideas and not the other way round.

Key Chapter Concepts

- Preventative medicine is predestined to play an increasingly important role in veterinary practices, both from a medical and business perspective.
- Current levels of compliance in our patients in the different areas of health are well below what we think. The main obstacle is not so much client resistance as failures in diagnostic protocols and monitoring by vets.
- To really boost preventive medicine in our practice we have to believe in it. We must rigorously complete clinical histories for all our patients, assume the role of client educators and devote time to measuring things.
- There are numerous examples of health plans or preventative medicine programmes that we can adapt for our practice. The real challenge lies not so much in the design of these programmes as in their efficient, rigorous and systematic implementation in our practice.

References

1. AAHA, Hill's. The Path to High-Quality Care, Practical Tips for Improving Compliance. 2003.
2. AVEPA, Hill's. Healthy Pets Mean Healthy Business, How Increased Compliance Makes Good Sense in Building a Modern, Caring Veterinary Practice. 2007.
3. With special thanks to the Hospital Veterinari del Maresme (Pere Guitart) for generously sharing this programme example.